Diagnosis: Cancer!

What happens next?

Gauri Bhide, M.D.

Copyright © 2018 Gauri Bhide, M.D.

All rights reserved. Except as permitted by the U.S. Copyright Act of 1976. No part of this publication may be reproduced, distributed or transmitted in any form or by any means, or stored in a database or retrieval system, without the prior written permission of the publisher.

The author has drawn all illustrations, except where attributed as instructed.Photographs were obtained from open source public domain images.

Fortitude Publishing House
http://www.fortitudepublishinghouse.com
fortitudepublishinghouse@gmail.com

First Edition January 2018
ISBN: 978-0-9983673-0-9

Dr. Gauri Bhide has created an accessible, readable, and highly informative guide that walks people through those first confusing weeks and months following a cancer diagnosis. As a psychologist whose research focuses on patient communication, and as a person who has been through ovarian cancer, I particularly appreciated Dr. Bhide's clear explanations of common cancer medical terms, treatment options, and her perspective not only as an oncologist, but as a wife of a person who went through cancer as she wrote the book. Like having a trusted friend who happens to be an oncologist walking through the maze of cancer treatment by ones' side, this book is an invaluable resource.

Karen Postal, Ph.D., ABPP
Board Certified Neuropsychologist
Lecturer, Harvard Medical School,
Boston, MA.

Patients with cancer are afforded many more options today in regards to treatments. While this has improved overall survival and quality of life, at times, the decision-making process can be overwhelming. With this book, Dr. Bhide provides a clear and comprehensive format in which patients are guided through the myriad of options available to them. In an easy-to-read style she takes patients from diagnosis, though treatment, to survivorship and, if needed, to end-of-life decision making. Even with 40 years of oncology experience, either as a patient or family member, I would find this book extremely helpful .

Fredrica Preston, N.P.
Massachusetts General Hospital, Boston, MA.

To the memory of
my parents,
who inspired me by their
resilience, persistence
and hard work.

Table of Contents

Section E: Beyond The Treatment

Section F:

Section G: Appendices

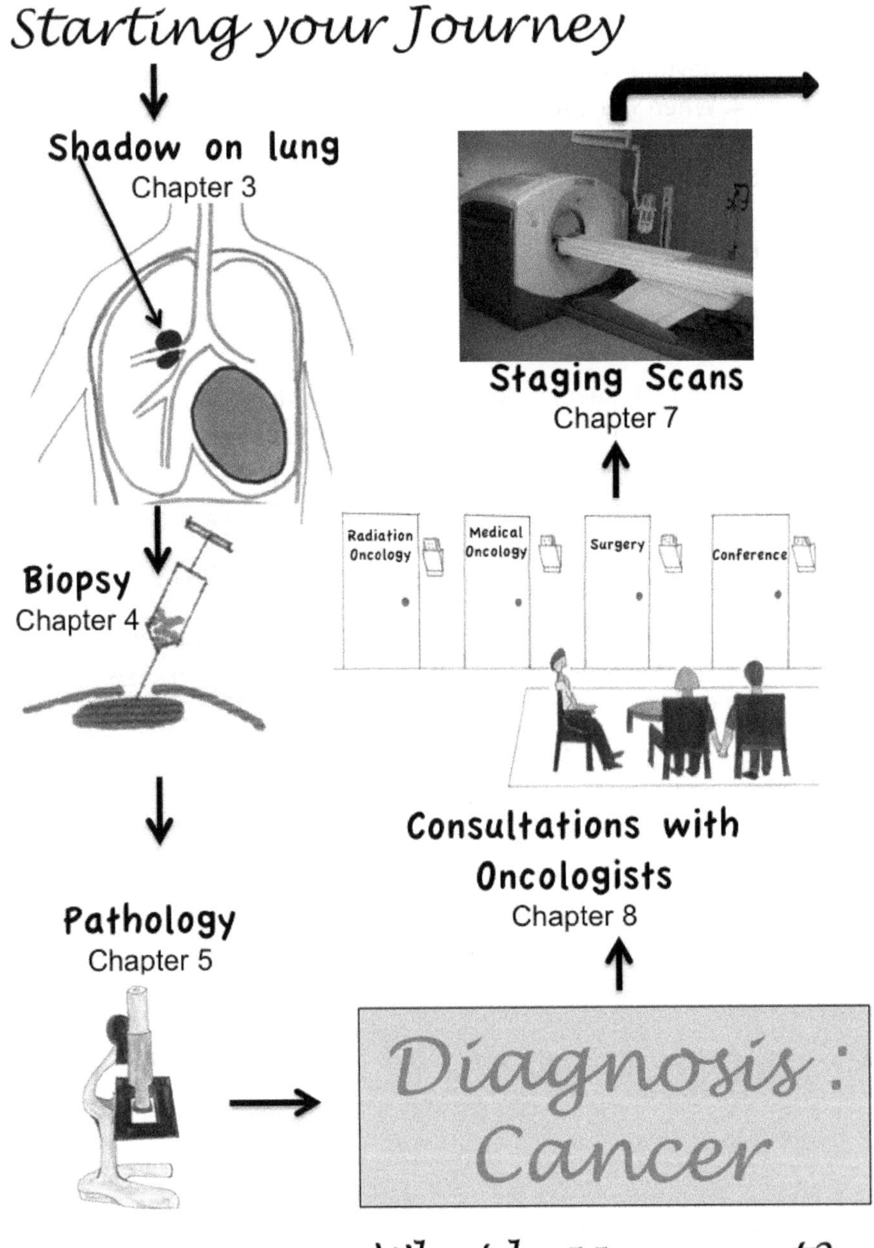

What happens next?

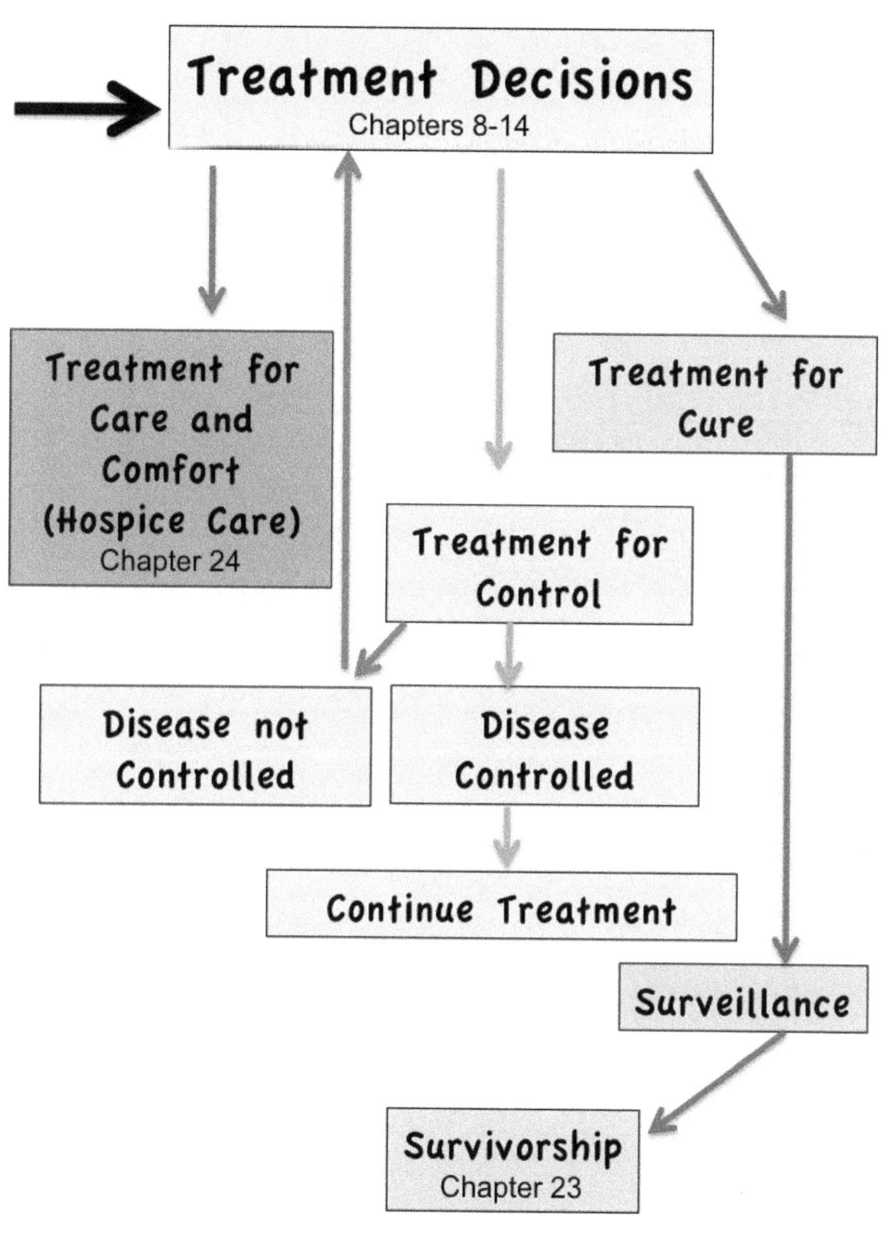

Decision Points along the way...

Foreword

So often, when patients first hear that they have cancer, they are immediately given a lot of information–sometimes from a lot of different doctors & nurses–and this can be very confusing.

I've been an oncology nurse for over thirty years, and I've worked in different types of Cancer Centers in four different states (including City of Hope, Dana Farber Cancer Center, and Memorial Sloan Kettering Cancer Center). I've taken care of many patients and worked with physicians, nurses, social workers and dietitians. And I'm a cancer survivor.

Sometimes there are different ways to treat cancer–perhaps surgery or chemotherapy or radiation therapy. Sometimes a combination of two of these treatments is recommended, and sometimes the best chance of a cure is for patients to be treated with all three types of treatment. Patients will be asked to make decisions about these various treatments, and these decisions may need to be taken fairly quickly-especially if it's best to start the treatment right away. Cancer is a chronic or long term disease, and it's a family disease–in other words it affects the patient and everyone who cares about the patient. And it is often years until treatment and follow up is finished.

Over the years I've noticed that when patients and loved ones have a better understanding of their illness and treatment they are not as worried or afraid. And when patients know more, they usually feel better asking questions. This makes it easier for them to make decisions about their care. When patients know what to expect while they are being treated, it helps them to be more relaxed.

This is why Dr. Gauri Bhide decided to write this book. It is for patients and their loved ones written in an easy-to-understand, conversational style. It is not meant to be another text book. It is for you, the patient, and your family and friends.

I first met Dr. Bhide about twenty years ago when we worked together at a community cancer center in Massachusetts. Although we no longer work together, my friendship with Dr. Bhide has continued. As well as being a highly skilled oncologist (cancer doctor) Dr. Bhide has always taken time to carefully explain everything she can about a patient's cancer diagnosis and treatment both to her patients and their loved ones. She has a passion for making sure that patients understand what is happening to their body, as well as their treatment options, the possible outcomes of treatment, and the side effects of treatment.

This book is a wonderful resource, and I believe that it will help you to learn more about cancer and its treatment as you start your journey. It will also help you to know what questions to ask when you see your doctors and nurses. Most importantly, it will help to take away some of the fear that goes along with hearing the words "You have cancer."

Gay Bailey, R.N., M.B.A.

Preface

Every Cancer patient and family is different...

As a Medical Oncologist I have had the opportunity of taking care of a variety of patients in all stages of cancer and across several countries. In different cultures patients and their families handle health issues differently. These global differences and preferences have made me sensitive to my patients' needs. Some patients need to understand everything that is going on and why; others prefer to hear the treatment decision directly. Some involve their families; others keep their illness very private. Some elderly patients make their own decisions; others rely on their children to help them decide. Some families from traditional cultures do not want to mention the word "cancer" to their parents believing it would be harmful to their mental health. In Western cultures autonomy and privacy in medical care is paramount. In other cultures patients often ask their doctors or family to make the medical decisions. It is important to take these factors into account in addition to providing good medical care.

Good listening and communication are key...

My patients have taught me the importance of good listening to both their spoken word and their body language, in order to insure that their needs are met. Specific situations have helped me crystalize my understanding of what cancer patients need. I will use many patient stories throughout this book to help illustrate the issues I am discussing although all names have been changed to protect patient privacy.

Here are some examples.

Lisa had completed her surgical treatment for breast cancer. Because of the stage of her cancer, she needed post-operative chemotherapy. Before starting chemotherapy she had been told that her treatment plan would consist of two phases. She had completed the first phase of four harsh treatments uneventfully, but she was having a difficult time with the transition to the second four that were going to be relatively easier treatments.

In spite of my various explanations, I was unable to soothe her anxiety. I listened hard to see what she needed from me. It became apparent that the main chemotherapy teaching session had been three months earlier, and the information she had been given about the second set of treatments had not registered. Once we arranged for a mini-teaching session, her anxiety abated. If we had not understood what she needed, her anxiety would have continued and might have affected how she reacted to the next round of treatments.

Because of this patient's experience, we started offering mini-teaching sessions to all patients who were transitioning from one phase of treatment to the next, even if we had covered the material in a previous teaching session. Not all patients took us up on it, but Lisa was happy that the breakthrough in our communication would help others.

*****

Judy came to me in great distress because of a newly diagnosed Stage 1 Breast Cancer. The specialist she had seen initially informed her that her Cancer was aggressive, recommended 6 months of chemotherapy as a precaution against a recurrence, and quoted a lot of scary numbers. Judy was on the verge doing no chemotherapy. The specialist had frightened her so much that she felt it was hopeless to try. As we talked, I reassured her that while her cell type was aggressive, her stage was still Stage 1. I offered to start with the first four chemotherapy treatments and reassess whether she wanted to do the next four after that. She readily agreed. At the end of the first four treatments, she decided against the next four, and she remains well ten years later.

*****

Dina was resisting the recommended chemotherapy having been told that it would affect the bone marrow. She was afraid it would worsen her osteoporosis. In reality, the bony part that is susceptible to osteoporosis surrounds the bone marrow and is not affected by chemotherapy. I realized her confusion and clarified the difference. She was satisfied and accepted the recommended chemotherapy.

Examples of such misunderstandings and confusion occur daily. Our patients are dealing with new and complicated medical language in addition to financial and emotional issues. It is very important to me that patients understand *why, how*, and *what* they are going to go through and that they participate in the decision-making. "Doctor speak" is very often confusing. We have to *listen*, to figure out what our patients don't understand, and be able to *explain it again*, until they *do* understand. Cancer treatment is a joint effort among the patient, their family, and the medical team. The doctor must understand what the patient needs, and the patient must understand what the doctor is saying. Miscommunication can cause misunderstanding and stress that can lead to a less than optimal outcome.

My motivation...

While I was writing this book, my husband was diagnosed with cancer. In spite of the shock, but because of my knowledge base, we understood what was happening, and we were able to navigate the process with more comfort. Surgery removed the tumor, and we are hopeful about a good long-term outcome.

While in the hospital, my husband's roommate, who was also newly diagnosed with cancer, had a number of questions and was frustrated when he could not get answers. The emotional and physical pain that he was experiencing was compounded by the frustration. I have helped friends and relatives deal with their diagnosis and treatment questions--acting as their coach. Over the years these calls have inspired me to bring this information to people who need it at the time they need it. Information is available on various websites, but the search can be confusing, overwhelming, time consuming, misleading, and full of "doctor speak." I want to bring this information to patients in one place in a format that will be helpful.

I sincerely hope it helps you.

Gauri Bhide, M.D.

DISCLAIMER

- The material presented in this book is for your information and education. It will provide a starting point for your understanding of your cancer. It is NOT a substitute for medical advice. Treatment options are changing with increasing rapidity. It is **vital** that you make your treatment decisions in consultation with your own medical team who can evaluate your individual situation.

Section A

Laying The Foundation

"To take care of cancer patients is an enormous privilege, but it also involves deploying everything in your toolbox: the emotional, the psychological, the scientific, the epidemiologic."

Siddhartha Mukherjee, M.D, D.Phil.
Author, Scientist, Oncologist.

1. How Will This Book Help You?

The words that change your life forever...

How did you get entangled in the web that cancer weaves? Your life has been turned upside down by the phone call that no one wants to get:

"Your X ray showed a suspicious mass and we need to do more tests." OR "Your biopsy showed cancer cells, and I'm going to send you to an Oncologist."

These words will change your life forever. This happened to us when my husband got that phone call. An ultrasound on Friday evening resulted in an entirely unexpected call from his Primary care doctor on Monday morning. I happened to be at home, and because of my experience as an Oncologist, we were able to get through the next few weeks until he completed his treatment.

I had already begun writing this book to guide patients with newly diagnosed cancer when we got this phone call. It now became a more personal mission to bring this information to others faced with a cancer diagnosis.

I'm sorry, but your X ray showed a shadow. We need to do more tests and send you to a specialist

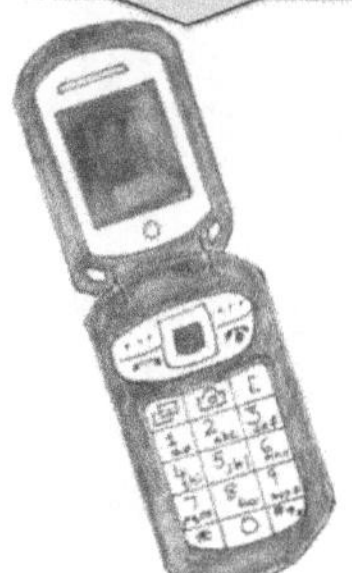

Figure 1.1

You've just been diagnosed with Cancer. What happens next?

If you or a family member has just been diagnosed with cancer, you feel as if you've been run over by a truck. Now what? Your mind is overrun with a million questions.

In today's information age, you can run to the computer and do an information search. But you soon discover all these unfamiliar terms. What does Stage mean? What does Grade mean? Why are there so many treatment choices? Why can't the doctors just cut it out? The surgeon said they got it all. Why do I need chemotherapy? Why do I need both radiation and chemotherapy? These are only some of the questions that will concern you.

The impact of a cancer diagnosis differs at different ages and in different family situations. If you are young and have a family or spouse to look after, you wonder, "Will I live long enough to see my children grow up? Will my spouse be a single parent? How will he/ she cope? How do I tell my children; what do I tell my children?"

If your children have grown up, you still think, "How do I tell my children." In addition, your family might have their own opinions on what you should do. They might pull you, the patient, in different directions because of how they are reacting to the news. Taking care of the medical and emotional issues, while at the same time figuring out how to manage the social and financial problems, is a balancing act.

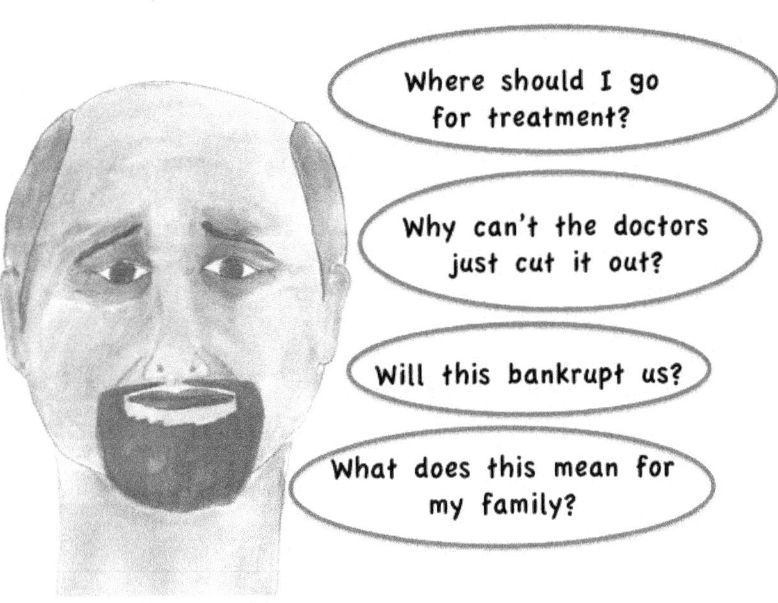

Figure 1.2

Cancer affects not just you...

Cancer affects the *whole* family *emotionally* with the fear of losing you and *financially* if you are unable to work for a while and they are dependent on your income. Grown-up children are torn between helping you and taking care of their own families. They may have to take time off from their jobs to come to your appointments or take you to your treatments. They are pulled in different directions: their jobs, their family, and you. It can also affect their own sense of mortality because they are afraid that they may now be at greater risk of developing cancer.

I don't understand the words. What do they mean? What are they talking about?

Medical professionals use technical terms that *they* use all the time thinking that those words are part of normal English language. Words in the medical language can have different meanings in everyday spoken language. Doctors don't realize that words we use routinely in a specific context can have an entirely different meaning for patients and their families. For example, we use the word *"invasive cancer"* in a very specific technical context. For the patient, however, the word *invasive* suggests whole body invasion. We will

Why me?
What does Stage mean?
What does grade mean?
What are my treatment options?
How long do I have?

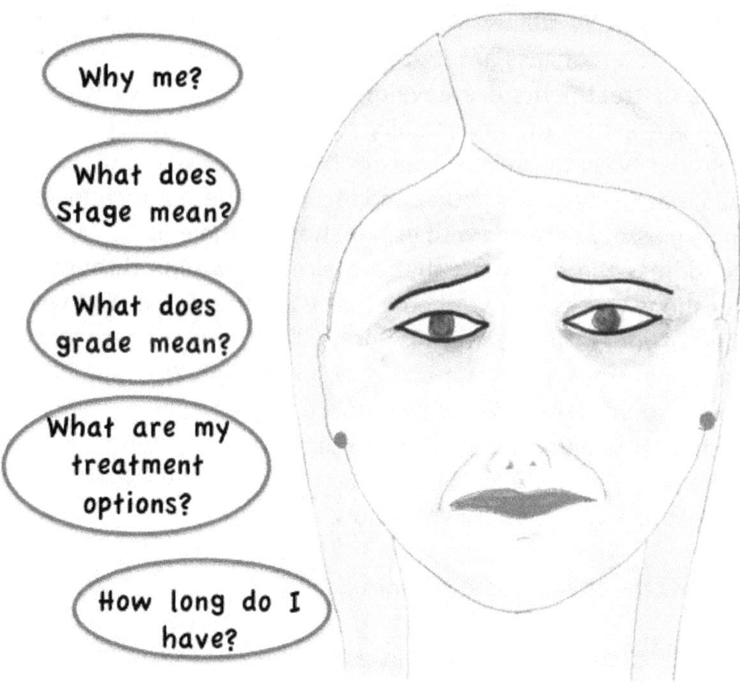

Figure 1.3

discuss invasion further in Chapter (5) when we discuss the Pathology report.

By the time I see patients for their first Oncology consultation (see Chapter 6), they have searched several websites, and they arrive in my office with a pile of printouts, many of which are not relevant to their *own* situation. In addition, they have usually received conflicting information and advice. Over the years I have addressed these questions through lengthy conversations with my patients. My mission? Patients and their families need to understand and be comfortable with their treatment choices. As you develop a good relationship with your Oncologist and your medical team, you should have ongoing conversations about the goals of your treatment plan and your needs and wishes.

So how will this book help you?

We will follow *Neal* - a patient diagnosed with lung cancer. We will meet him in Chapter 3 when he is admitted to the hospital with pneumonia. By following Neal's journey from *diagnosis to treatment*, this book will walk you through the information you will need to get through your own diagnosis, treatment, and beyond. The first few chapters will help you understand the difference between a normal cell and the cancer cell and will introduce the vocabulary that will be used in future chapters. Chapters on treatment and supportive care follow. Then we will discuss the way clinical trials are conducted, how statistics are used to evaluate cancer treatments, and how standards of treatments are developed. When you finish with treatment, you may face issues of survivorship, so we will talk about those. We will also consider ways to prevent cancer. Many checklists and worksheets are included that will help you gather and record the necessary information. You will find a glossary of terms with explanations at the end.

I will address the questions that are already swirling through your mind and questions you do not yet know that you should ask. You will meet the members of your future team. This book will help you prepare for your future visits and the procedures that you may go through. We will talk about the available resources that will help you through your treatments.

Each chapter will end with an action plan and questions to ask your team along the way. You can read through the chapters sequentially or skip ahead to the ones that you need the most now.

Here is how the chapters are organized:

Chapter 1 illustrates possible scenarios that may have brought you to this diagnosis.

Chapter 2 describes the basic structure of a cell and considers how a normal cell becomes a cancer cell.
Chapters 3 and 4 explain the process of making a cancer diagnosis.
Chapter 5 will interpret the Pathology report.
Chapter 6 gives helpful hints on how to get the most out of your consultations.
Chapter 7 will explain what Staging means and why it is needed.
Chapters 8 to 14 talk about treatment choices and discuss treatment related issues.
Chapters 15 to 18 deal with practical questions of general advice, fertility, nutrition and genetics.
Chapters 19 and 20 discuss Complementary Therapy and the Mind-Body Connection.
Chapters 21 and 22 describe how clinical trials are developed and how treatments are evaluated.
Chapter 23 deals with survivorship issues.
Chapter 24 addresses your option of foregoing treatment and focusing simply on care and comfort.
The Appendices describe common medicines you may be prescribed along with checklists and work sheets. Much of this information, especially on cancer prevention and screening, may be of assistance to your entire family. At the end is a list of reliable resources to which you can refer.

Who are the Specialists who treat cancer?

- **Radiation Oncologist:** Doctor who treats cancer with radiation therapy.
- **Medical Oncologist:** Doctor who treats cancer with chemotherapy, hormone therapy, targeted agents or immunotherapy.
- **Cancer Surgeon:** Surgeon who specializes in cancer surgery.
- **Hematologist:** Doctor who treats blood disorders. Blood disorders can be a bone marrow cancer like leukemia OR disorders like anemia or bleeding and clotting problems that are not cancers.

Often, specialists train in both Medical Oncology and Hematology and see both these categories of diseases. You may see a doctor in a Cancer Center for a benign anemia like an anemia related to iron or vitamin deficiency. Seeing the doctor in the Cancer Center does not mean you have cancer.

ACTION PLAN

- Don't jump to conclusions. Wait until you get all your results.
- Be aware that web searches may not yield reliable information.
- Start making " healthful choices": eat better, exercise and quit smoking.
- Get an agenda book or diary to keep track of your appointments and information.
- Read this book to prepare for your visits and as your guide to treatment.
- Make notes as you go along.

2. What Is Cancer?

How do tumors start, grow and spread?

The word cancer evokes fear and dread because we have all seen the destruction it causes in the human body. But what is a cancer cell? Where does it come from? How does it grow and spread and why does it cause death? Many lay people think that we are all born with cancer cells and that they grow in some people but not in others. Let us address these questions. The explanation for some of these questions may be technical, but it will help you understand your disease and treatment choices. If you feel you are not ready for so much explanation, you may reserve this chapter for a later date.

Firstly we should consider just what is a cell?

The cell is the basic unit in our body. It is bound by a cell membrane and contains cytoplasm and a nucleus. At the center is the nucleus which is the brain of the cell and contains the chromosomes that carry genes. Genes contain the DNA code which determines both how we function and which characteristics we pass on to our offspring. The cytoplasm is the body of the cell; in addition to the nucleus it contains many packages of energy (mitochondria) and other housekeeping material. The cell is outlined by the cell membrane. Nutrients, the food that keeps the cell alive, enter the cell through special channels in the cell membrane. Cells cluster in groups,

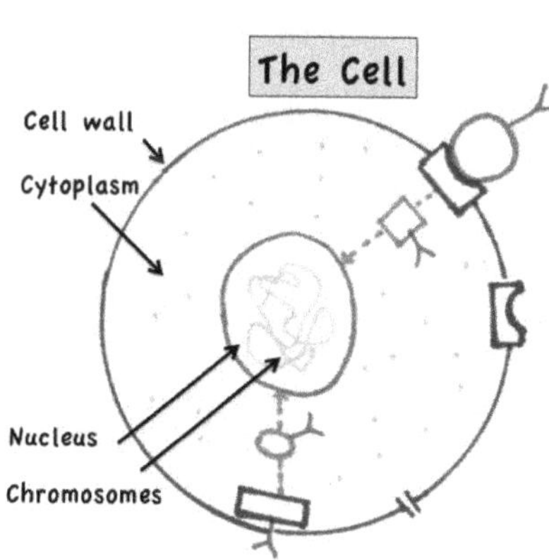

Figure 2.1

and they communicate with their neighbors and environment through special receptors or gateways. Different messengers, like hormones, bind to their own unique receptors on the cell surface. This binding is like a secret handshake. It sends a signal to the nucleus and tells the cell to change or grow in an orderly and controlled fashion.

Groups of cells are organized into different tissues, which have different functions. For example, some tissues form glands that secrete digestive enzymes. That tissue is then organized into a digestive organ, for example the stomach, into which the glands send the enzymes to digest our food. Organs are grouped into organ systems like the digestive system, or circulatory system. All these systems are both interconnected and interdependent and work together to help the body function as a whole.

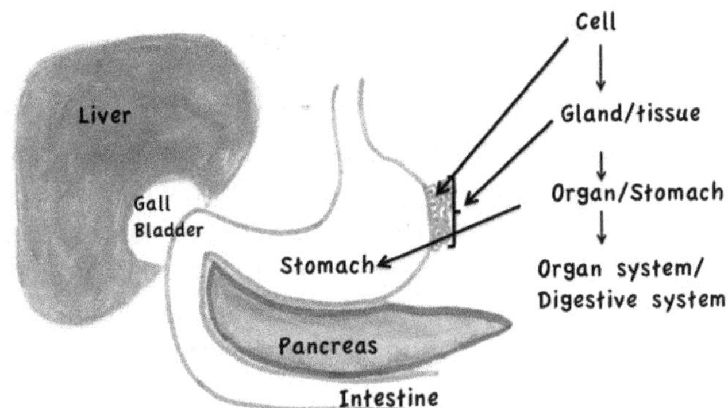

Figure 2.2

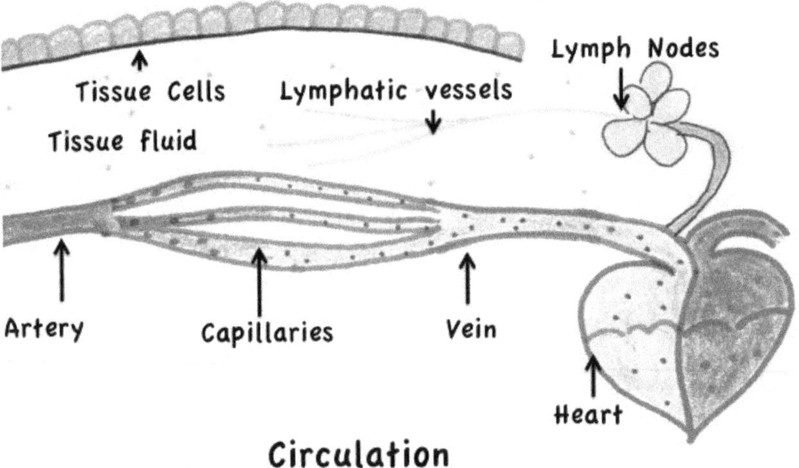

Figure 2.4

Nutrients that the tissues need to live are brought to them by blood vessels called arteries. Blood flows back into circulation via capillaries and veins. The tissue is bathed in tissue fluid that is then drained by lymph vessels (or lymphatics). The main roads in and out of town are like blood vessels (arteries and veins). Streets that run through the neighborhoods are like capillaries and lymph vessels.

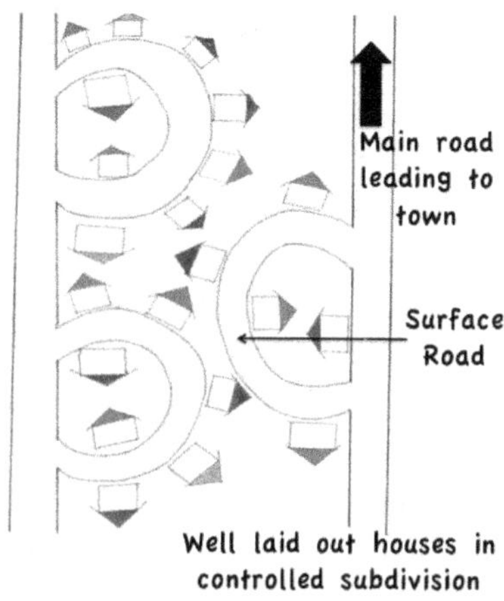

Figure 2.3

One way of describing this organization is to think of each cell as a house. A collection of houses forms a subdivision or a neighborhood. A collection of subdivisions makes a town in the same way as a specialized collection of tissues create a specific organ.

Cell-->Tissue-->Organ =
House-->subdivision-->Town

In time houses get old and need to be repaired or torn down. Normal cells also age and die out. This is accomplished in our bodies in an internally pre-programmed manner. Old cells die and new ones take their place in a controlled manner. Different cells have different replacement rates. Some kinds of cells are replaced every few days and others every few months. Some special kinds of cells are never replaced. Heart muscle cells, for example, are not replaced after a heart attack.

Are we all born with cancer cells?

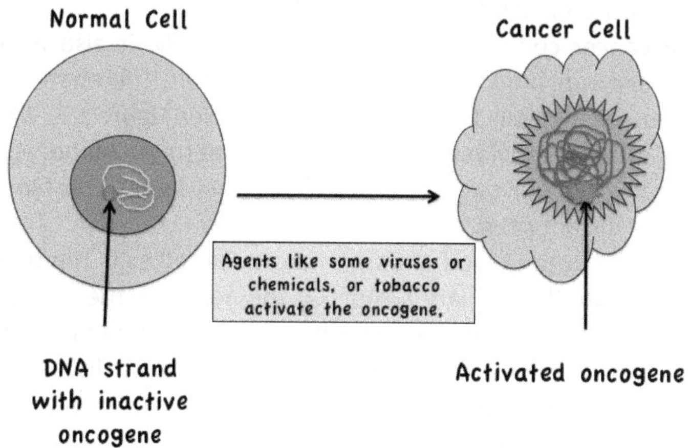

Figure 2.5

We are not actually born with cancer cells. All dividing cells, however, have the potential to become cancerous. 'Proto-oncogenes,' or genes that can transform the cell into a cancer cell when activated into oncogenes, are found in the nucleus of normal cells. There are also tumor-suppressor genes that usually overcome the tumor-promoting genes. If the tumor-suppressor gene loses the battle, the activated oncogene allows the cells to divide uncontrollably and spread. Normally, when such "mistakes" or cancerous changes occur, the immune system recognizes the abnormal cell as "not self" and destroys it, like a scavenging system or a "clean up brigade."

Cancer cells survive when the cell loses its normal internal control mechanism *and* escapes detection by the clean-up brigade. Exposure to environmental toxins or the chemicals in tobacco smoke can affect the internal signaling pathway of the cell. This "liberates" the cell from the normal control mechanism and can lead to cancer.

How do tumors form from normal tissue?

As we said above, when cells get old and die, the body replaces them continuously in a *controlled* manner. When this internal control system goes wrong and the cells do not die as they should. They continue to divide and accumulate to cause a tumor or a lump. Some tumors form lumps under the skin and you can feel them. Others are inside the body and show up only in scans.

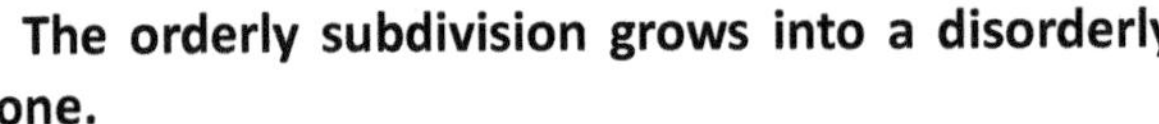

The orderly subdivision grows into a disorderly one.

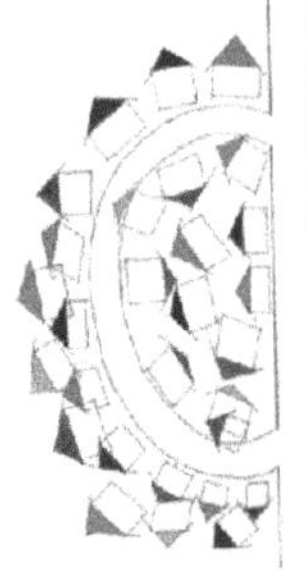

Overcrowded and uncontrolled subdivision

Figure 2.6

How does a cancer grow and spread?

When the cancer cell starts *dividing uncontrollably*, it also acquires the capacity to *penetrate* blood vessels and lymph vessels. This enables cancer to *spread* to vital organs away from the original site. (See Figure 2.7) A cancerous tumor does all three: divides uncontrollably, penetrates blood vessels, and spreads. A benign tumor cell only divides; it neither penetrates blood vessels nor spreads to distant sites.

After circulating in the blood stream, the cancer cell exits the blood vessel at a site away from the primary tumor. At the new site, the cancer cell gets busy. It grows, divides, seeds the development of new tumors, attracts blood vessels, and starts occupying the organ. The new site of disease is called a Metastasis or a Secondary site. Metastases occur commonly in the liver, bones, lungs, and brain. (See Figure 2.8)

What is a Lymph Node?

Lymph, or tissue fluid, bathes the cells and is necessary for exchange of nutrients. It is carried away from the tissues by lymphatics. Eventually this fluid is directed back into the blood stream for circulation. Before it gets there it passes through a collection of immunity processing cells which check for foreign antigens and produce antibodies to fight infection. These lymph nodes act as service stations, processing antibodies to fight infection, and are located along the lymphatic circulatory system. Each body part has its own service station. (See Figure 2.9). An example is the glands in your neck which swell when you have a sore throat. They are helping fight the infection in your throat. When there is cancer in a Primary site, the cancer cell can travel to the local lymph nodes, and that provides a gateway to the rest of the body. If the lymph nodes do not have cancer cells, they are unlikely to have spread further.

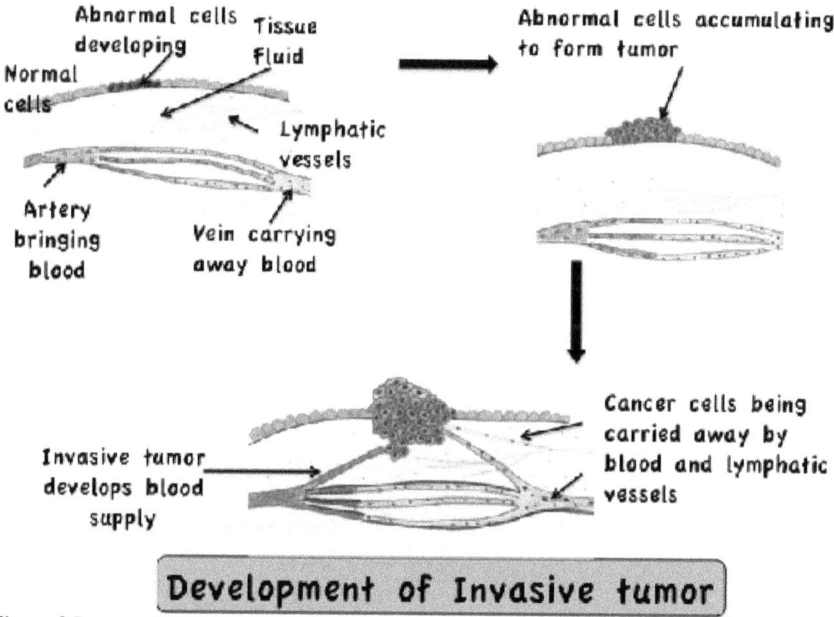

Figure 2.7

Are all lumps or tumors cancerous?

Not all lumps or tumors are cancerous (or malignant). A lump can be benign: it grows locally; it doesn't spread; it is not lethal. For example, a collection of benign fibrous tissue is called a fibroma. A collection of benign fatty tissue is called a lipoma. Sometimes a mixture of different types of cells makes a fibro-adenoma which is a common type of benign breast lump. Benign tumors contain normal cells accumulated in an abnormal quantity. They do not invade blood vessels and travel. Other than their sometimes unpleasant physical presence, they do not cause ill effects. They can be small, like moles, or they can grow to a substantial size and cause discomfort locally by pressing on a blood vessel or nerve.

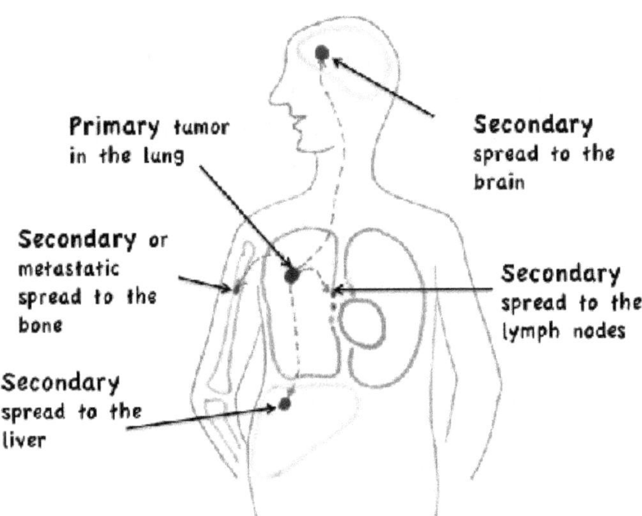

Figure 2.8

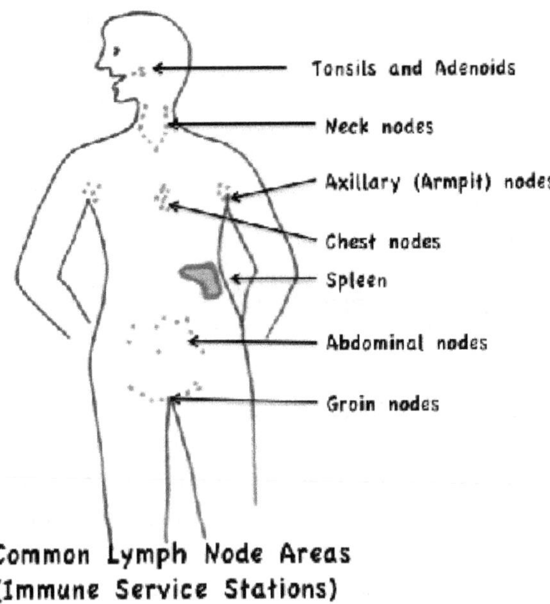

Figure 2.9

How do you tell if a lump is benign or cancerous?

"I have a lump in my breast. The doctors say they don't need to take it out. They say it is not cancer." Some benign tumors need to biopsied or even removed to make sure they are not cancerous. Others, if they have no suspicious characteristics of a cancer and can be easily observed for any changes, do not. If the doctors have been following you for similar lumps, and have biopsied a similar lump, they may not need to biopsy this one.

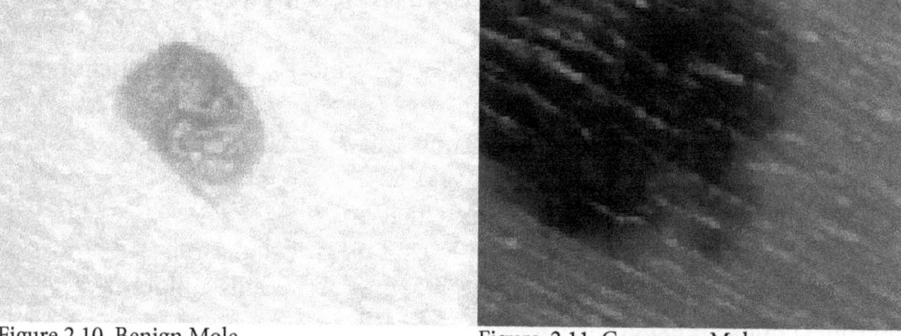

Figure 2.10 Benign Mole

Figure 2.11 Cancerous Mole.

How does Cancer cause death?

Death results from cancer in several ways. The Primary tumor or the Secondary metastasis grows and eats away at the vital organs. Cancer cells also produce chemicals called cytokines which have many ways of making a person feel ill including loss of appetite, weight loss, fatigue, and fevers. Imagine a residential neighborhood being "invaded" by one cement factory, then another, and another. Soon the neighborhood is taken over by an industrial complex complete with industrial waste products and heavy traffic. Residents lose out to the factories. The normal organ loses out to the invading cancer.

Why did this happen to me?

"Uncle Joe smoked like a chimney, and he died of old age. I never smoked, why did I get Lung Cancer? "

"Cancer doesn't run in my family, so why did I get it?"

There are no straightforward answers to these questions because cancer occurs for many reasons, and a series of events is usually the cause.

In some cases **inherited or accidental mutations**, or faulty genes, can affect the body's ability to correct mistakes. Some mutations will predispose a person to only one kind of cancer; others can predispose a person to a group of cancers. Some cancers require only one mistake, but others need a sequence of mistakes.

Toxins in our environment like the industrial solvent benzene cause chronic irritation. Radiation from nuclear accidents can cause acute toxic injury and also lead to cancer-causing genetic mutations. Radon gas leaks out of the earth and into the basements of homes, and chronic exposure to Radon can cause lung cancer. The many cancer-causing chemicals in tobacco smoke constantly coat the air passages with each inhalation, and this chronic irritation can lead to cancerous changes.

Viruses like HPV (human papilloma virus) can cause changes in the lining of the female cervix and initiate the process leading to cancer. HPV is also implicated in cancers of the throat. EBV (Epstein Barr virus) infection can contribute to some lymphomas or cancers of the lymph glands. Chronic viral infections of the liver with Hepatitis B and C can lead to liver cancers.

Why did this happen to you? Why not Uncle Joe?

Our body's immune system efficiently gets rid of cellular mistakes most of the time, but it's not perfect. Everyone's body responds differently to the internal changes it experiences.

Sometimes mistakes survive because the irritants (e.g. cigarette smoke) were chronic and overwhelming. Sometimes a number of these events may have to occur before a tumor becomes cancerous. Not all smokers will get lung cancer, and not all people with inherited mutations will develop cancer. What separates the two? We do not know yet. Research continues, and we must be aware and decrease our personal risk factors as much as possible. You cannot change your genes, but you and your family can work on changing those lifestyles that can contribute to cancer. Having a family member get cancer can be a motivating factor to give up smoking, eat right, start exercising, and lose weight.

Examples of risk factors that contribute to Cancers

- Environment: Chemicals, radiation, viruses.
- Genes: Inherited mutations.
- Habits: Tobacco use (smoking, or chewing), excess alcohol, excess weight, dietary habits.

Action Plan

- Avoid cancer-causing habits, mainly tobacco use.
- Limit alcohol, fats and red meat. Eat more fruits and vegetables.
- Exercise. Maintain a normal BMI.
- Use antiviral vaccines when appropriate: Hepatitis, HPV.
- Know your family cancer history.
- Follow recommended screening guidelines.

Glossary

- HPV= Human Papilloma Virus.
- EBV= Epstein Barr Virus.
- Primary site= Originating point of tumor.
- Metastasis or Secondary site= Disease away from the Primary site.
- Mutation=Change in gene or protein structure affecting function.
- BMI= Body Mass Index, is a measure of obesity.

Section B

The Path To A Cancer Diagnosis

"If one does not know to which port one is sailing, no wind is favorable."

Lucius Annaeus Seneca
Roman Philosopher

3. From Symptoms to Diagnosis

What led to your diagnosis?

In this chapter we will meet several patients who were diagnosed with cancer in different scenarios. We especially will meet Neal, and then we will follow his journey from his symptoms through his treatment. While his journey may be different from yours, we will review the information that you will need for your own treatment decisions.

Sometimes we do not experience any symptoms and cancer shows up on the recommended screening tests. At other times we know something is not right but haven't had time to look into it. Perhaps a doctor's appointment is coming up in a couple of months, and it seems OK to wait until then. Occasionally a scan is done for a different purpose but picks up a tumor that was not causing any symptoms yet. Perhaps one of these following scenarios is similar to yours.

How do we find Cancers in the early Stages?

Anita was really good about keeping up with her mammograms. Her mother's sister had had breast cancer in her 50s, and Anita was very aware of the importance of screening tests. When she turned 50, her primary doctor discussed the importance of another kind of screening test-- a colonoscopy. This involves doing a bowel cleanse and then having a flexible tube containing a light inserted into the rectum and passed up through the colon to look for internal polyps. If any are found, they can be removed right away which will prevent them from turning into colon cancer. No one in her family had colon cancer, but Anita readily agreed. That turned out to be a wise move. A few small polyps were developing in her large intestine, and one had a speck of cancer at its tip. This was removed in its entirety, and she was cured.

Anita represents the success of Screening.

Follow Screening guidelines. These are provided in the Appendix.

Roger went to his Primary doctor for his annual checkup. His doctor had encouraged him for several years to lose weight. Roger had tried some diets, but he couldn't stick with them. He was tired at the end of a long day of work, and a salad didn't quite satisfy him. He tried to exercise regularly, but it was hard to keep it up with his schedule. He couldn't make any time to exercise. There was just too much to do. He was on his feet all day long, and all he wanted to do at the end of the day was grab a beer and catch the ball game on TV. He always dreaded facing the scale in his doctor's office, but this year he was looking forward to surprising his doctor. He just hadn't been as hungry for the last few months and wasn't finishing his dinner.

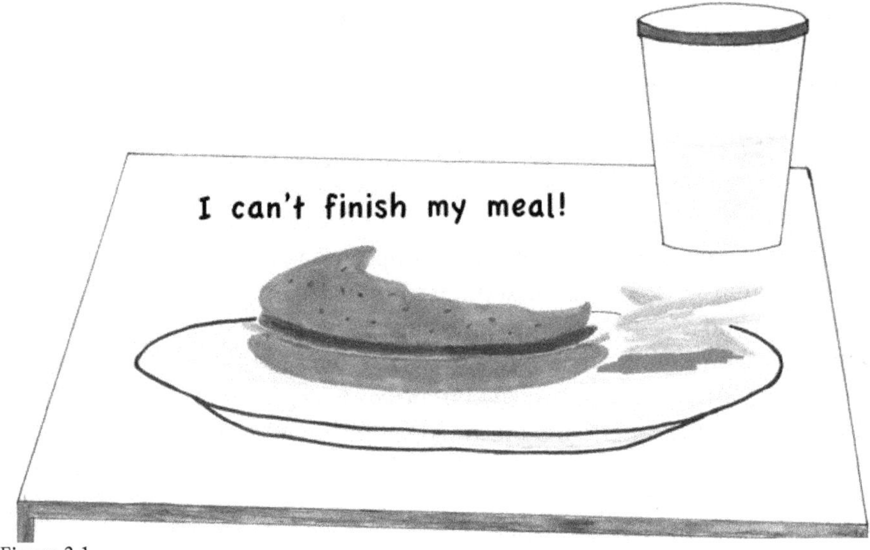

Figure 3.1

Roger was taking antacids more frequently, but he thought it was related to his new boss. The company was changing direction, and there was a lot of stress at work. Roger was feeling more rundown and was hoping his doctor could suggest some vitamins to give him some energy. He had meant to call the doctor a few months ago, but he just didn't make the time. He knew his annual physical was coming up and thought it could wait till then.

Doc: "Roger, I should be happy with your weight loss, but losing 25 pounds without trying doesn't sound good. Losing your appetite to that extent is not you. Are you having difficulty swallowing, or are you feeling full or bloated halfway through a meal? "

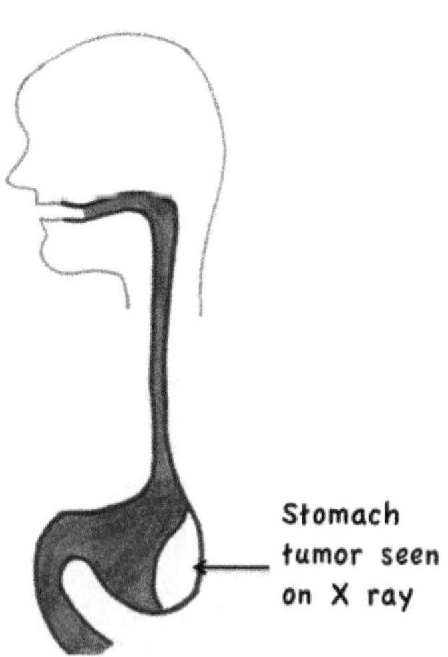

Figure 3.2

Roger: "Both. I can't finish my dinner most nights, and I feel full halfway through. I thought that was good--that it was helping me eat less. You keep talking to me about portion control."

Doc: "Well, yes. But I don't like how it is happening. Let's run some tests."

The doctor ordered an X ray study called an Upper GI (gastrointestinal) study. X rays were taken while Roger swallowed some white Barium solution to see if anything obstructed the flow of the Barium.

The Radiologist called Roger's doctor that day. There was something suspicious in Roger's stomach. CAT scans and an Upper Endoscopy confirmed that Roger had stomach cancer. The tumor that occupied his stomach had been preventing him from finishing his meals.

Roger's body had been telling him something, but he had been too stressed and too busy to listen.

Listen to your body. Report your symptoms.

Neal was a lifelong smoker. He had tried to quit smoking many times but couldn't last more than a week. He was used to spending some time every morning hacking and coughing, trying to bring up the phlegm that had accumulated overnight. Sometimes his phlegm contained specks of blood. Last year he had been hospitalized for pneumonia, and every winter he had a couple of bouts of bronchitis. This last week, when he couldn't catch his breath, he coughed up a dollop of blood. That scared him, and he went to the Emergency Room to see if he had developed pneumonia. A CT scan of his chest showed a big shadow behind his heart. The ER doctors admitted Neal to the hospital and looked into his airways the next morning. Unfortunately they found a tumor next to his airway, and the biopsy confirmed lung cancer.

Give feedback to your doctor.

Even if you have had similar symptoms before, when the symptoms get worse, go back to your doctor. If the antibiotics for a presumed infection don't help, go back to your doctor. Something else may be going on.

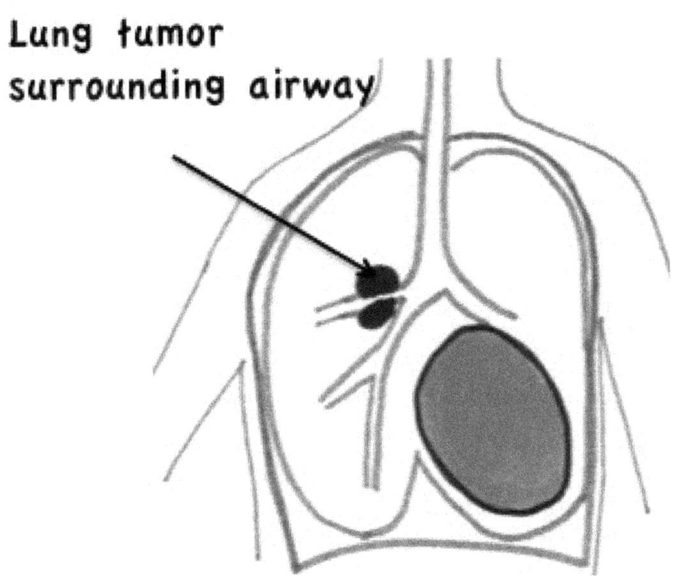

Figure 3.3

Both Neal and Roger found their disease after it had caused symptoms: pain, bleeding, inability to eat properly, weight loss, fatigue, inability to breathe easily, etc. These symptoms can be easily mistaken for regular heartburn, life stress, bronchitis, pneumonia, and irritable bowel disease—all of which are more common than cancer. The challenge is to recognize when the symptoms are too abnormal for a routine sickness and when to investigate more thoroughly.

What could Roger or Neal have done differently?

Both Neal and Roger could have called their doctors when they first noticed that something was really different. Even if a routine appointment is coming up in a month or two, a quick visit might see if the new symptoms are cause for concern. Often it is difficult for both the doctor and the patient to decide when a chronic problem like Neal's has become an actionable issue. Because it is a team effort, having a good relationship with your Primary doctor is key. It may take multiple visits to differentiate a cough from asthma or chronic bronchitis from a cough caused by lung cancer. Fatigue and unexplained weight loss may be your only symptoms.

Would earlier diagnosis have helped?

Roger and Neal's cancers were not diagnosed in an early stage for many reasons. Most cancers do not have screening tests and can only be diagnosed when they cause symptoms. Even if early diagnosis is desired, it is not always possible. The later the disease is diagnosed, however, the more chance it has to weaken your body. Acting on symptoms in a timely fashion can mean that the disease has not spread, there are more treatment options, and you have a better ability to successfully complete the treatment.

And then you can get lucky...

David had been feeling great. He had been found to have borderline high cholesterol and blood sugars at last year's check up, and he had been diligently exercising and watching his food intake. He was hoping this year's check up would show progress in his lipid and sugar levels, but they were still high. His doctor wanted to put him on pills for diabetes and high cholesterol. He ordered an ultrasound of his liver because his liver blood tests were also slightly abnormal. The ultrasound of David's liver was OK, but while looking at the liver, they found a mass on his kidney. They discovered this by accident since David had no complaints related to his kidneys. He was scheduled for surgery. As he said later, "Developing diabetes saved my life."

We hear of these situations, and we wonder what lurks in our bodies. Would it be worthwhile to get a full body scan? A few years ago some commercial outfits were marketing whole body scans as a precaution, but this practice has not been validated and is not one of the recommended screening tests. We will review issues on screening and the guidelines in the appendix of the book.

If cancer cells are hiding in my body, how can I find them? I was having blood tests with my check ups. Why didn't that find the cancer?

Routine blood tests with your annual checkups check for diabetes, cholesterol, kidney and liver function, thyroid function, and anemia. *No recommended blood test exists to screen for cancer.* A routine blood test for PSA (Prostate Specific Antigen) is controversial for screening for prostate cancer. Other blood tests (for example, CA-125 for ovarian cancer and CEA for colon cancer) are done *after* the cancer has been diagnosed to measure the response to treatment--not for early diagnosis. At this time no routine blood tests will find individual cancer cells. Ongoing research is trying to identify a method to detect circulating tumor cells (CTCs). If these methods are validated, they may add to the ability to detect cancer early.

There are screening procedures (not blood tests) that have been developed to find some cancers at an early stage. Finding cancer in the early stages can result in a cure, but there are established Screening procedures for specific cancers only, namely breast, colon, cervix and lung (in high risk smokers). For most cancers, the best approach is to be aware of changes in your body.

Many people fear that they will become hypochondriacs if they are too vigilant. There is a balance between being vigilant and being a hypochondriac.

Some Symptoms you should report:

- Unexplained weight loss or loss of appetite.
- Daily fevers, or fevers with sweats.
- Coughing blood, or passing blood in the urine or stools.
- Lumps that you can feel.
- Unexplained pain or swelling.
- Change in size or color of moles, or new skin lesions that will not heal.
- Difficulty swallowing or speaking.
- Change in your voice.
- Sores on your tongue or in your mouth.

Action Plan

- Follow Screening Guidelines.
- Listen to your body; do not avoid reporting bad signs.
- Give your doctor feedback if the first treatment doesn't work.
- Take care of your body: Exercise, Use alcohol in moderation, NEVER use tobacco.
- Eat fruits and vegetables daily; eat a healthy, balanced diet.

4. The Path to Diagnosis

We met *Neal* in Chapter 3. He was admitted to the hospital with pneumonia and was diagnosed with a lung tumor. There are many ways that cancer can show itself. You reported your symptoms and had some tests, OR you had your screening test which came back abnormal. This chapter will walk you through the process of making a diagnosis.

What happens next?

Whether it is by physical examination or by scans, something abnormal is noted. This is variously called a **lump, a shadow, a nodule, a mass or a tumor**, all of which means they see something that shouldn't be there. Until it is *proven* to be cancer by a biopsy, it is not called cancer. Cancer, however, needs to be considered in all abnormal shadows, lumps, or nodules. Some shadows are more suspicious for cancer than others and need a biopsy for further management right away. Some shadows are clearly not cancerous by established criteria. Doctors follow those with serial examinations or scans to make sure they don't change. Increase in size will increase the suspicion for cancer. At that point, you will need a biopsy.

It is important to note that the only way to diagnose cancer is by having a Pathologist examine cells that have been removed from the abnormal mass with a biopsy. A Pathologist is a doctor who specializes in identifying cells. Your treatment plan will be decided based on the Pathologist's findings.

What is a biopsy?

A biopsy is a sample of tissue taken from the abnormal spot, and there are a number of ways of getting to the tumor.

If your doctor felt a lump on physical examination, she can place a needle directly into it for a sample of cells. Sometimes the lump itself can be removed and sent to the Pathologist for microscopic tissue examination.

If the spot was seen on a mammogram or a CT scan, a sample is taken by repeating the scan. The spot is located while the patient is on the scanner table, and a needle is placed in that spot. Usually local anesthesia is sufficient for this procedure. Sometimes mild sedation may be added. This procedure does not involve an operation. A specially trained Radiologist called an Interventional Radiologist performs it, and this kind of biopsy can be done as an outpatient. You are kept for observation for a couple of hours afterward to make sure there are no delayed complications.

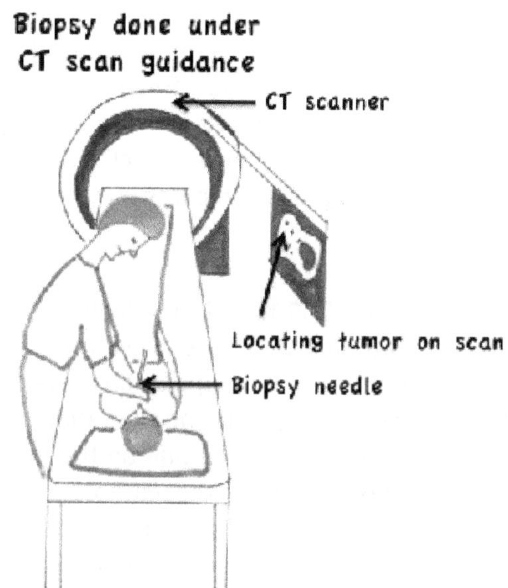

Figure 4.1

Sometimes the biopsy cannot be obtained safely in this manner either because the abnormal spot is too deep or it is too close to delicate organs. In that case a surgical procedure may be required.

If surgery is done *only* for the biopsy, the tissue is sampled and the further treatment will be undertaken after the results. If it is a *planned cancer operation*, a quick look (Frozen section: see below) by the Pathologist confirms cancer. Then the Surgeon will proceed with a full operation, and the tumor and additional tissue will be removed in its entirety.

A biopsy can also be done during a *colonoscopy,* which is a screening procedure for colon cancer. If a polyp or growth on the inside of the colon is found on a colonoscopy (direct examination of the inside of the colon) the polyp is removed during the colonoscopy and sent to the Pathologist. A *bronchoscopy* is a similar procedure but looks internally into your air passages. A *cystoscopy* involves looking inside your bladder. A sample of tissue can then be taken from any abnormal area.

What is the difference between an aspirate and a biopsy? My doctor already did an aspirate. Why do I need a biopsy?

An *aspirate* is often a smaller procedure and uses a skinny needle to aspirate or extract some cells to see if cancer cells are present. During this process the cells separate from each other. An aspirate gives us a Yes or No answer whether cancer cells are present. This is useful to confirm the presence of cancer particularly if the cancer is suspected in a Secondary site. To plan treatment, however, we will need additional information like the internal organization of the cancer cells, whether blood vessels have been invaded, or whether the capsule around the cancerous tumor has been penetrated. For this we need a full biopsy, which is a solid piece of tumor tissue to examine the internal organization of the cells. This is accomplished with a thicker needle. The tissue in the core of the needle is removed intact instead of sucking out the cells. This is called a *core biopsy.* Several cores may be taken to get adequate tissue for examination.

What happens next? Why does it take so long to get an answer?

The biopsy tissue is then sent to the Pathologist. It takes several days to process the tissue and do a thorough examination. If an operation was done, sometimes the Pathologist can take a quick look during the operation. This is called a "frozen section." This may help the Surgeon decide on the extent of surgery before completing the operation. Even if the Pathologist can say whether cancer cells are present, the tissue still needs to be properly processed for a detailed examination, and a full report will take a few days. If the biopsy was obtained by an external needle biopsy, a frozen section is usually not performed. The amount of tissue is small, and it needs to be processed to isolate the cells to be examined.

Two Pathologists usually examine the slides to confirm the diagnosis. Often the tissue is sent out to a specialty lab to perform additional tests for special proteins or receptors on the cell surface. The presence or absence of those proteins or receptors will help the Oncologist determine the kind of treatment. For example, the presence of estrogen receptors on the breast cancer cell will make hormone treatment an option. (See Chapter 9, Treatment Choices).

Genetic testing can also reveal the presence of mutations that can be a target for treatment. In fact, in the coming years, tests for gene mutations and receptor analysis may be more important in treatment planning than the organ of origin of the cancer. As you will read in Chapter 10 on treatment choices, we have already moved away from surgery as the primary treatment for most cancers. A combination of surgery, chemotherapy, or radiation therapy is often used. In the future, treatment directed against receptors and mutations may replace current methods of chemotherapy.

In some cancers additional gene testing on the tumor DNA can provide a score that can predict the risk for recurrence, for example the Oncotype Dx score in breast cancer. A high recurrence score justifies the use of preventive chemotherapy. A low recurrence score tells us you may not need chemotherapy.

Confirming the diagnosis and gathering all the relevant information is the most important part of the process. This is why it takes so long to get the answer. The waiting is difficult, but it is really important to get it right.

We will review the components of the Pathology report in Chapter 5.

Where was your cancer diagnosed? This will affect how the process moves from here on.

There are two main situations under which your cancer can be discovered: in the hospital (as an inpatient), or outside the hospital, as an outpatient.

In the Hospital...

Like Neal, John was admitted to the hospital for pneumonia. The doctor found a tumor in his lung, he had a biopsy, and he was going through a number of scans. He was seeing a lot of doctors, but no one was giving him a straight answer about treatment.

John was frustrated because he was admitted for pneumonia but then discovered he had a tumor. The doctors who were the consultants in the hospital could not definitely tell him how he was going to be treated for his cancer. They would only speak in general terms. The consultants in the hospital were guiding the care until he got discharged. He couldn't meet the doctors who would eventually take care of his cancer while he was in the hospital. He wanted them all to confer and give him their opinion now, while he was in the hospital.

If you are hospitalized for the symptom that led to your diagnosis, for instance a pneumonia that unmasked a lung cancer, or intestinal blockage that revealed a hidden colon cancer, the doctors in the hospital (known as Hospitalists) manage your care for the problem for which you were admitted to the hospital. They consult an Oncologist to help them guide the investigation for the cancer, and they take care of the immediate situation like the pneumonia or the intestinal blockage. They will eventually hand over your care to the appropriate specialist when you are discharged from the hospital.

It may seem like you are seeing too many different specialists and repeating your story to too many different people. In most large Centers, however, care has become compartmentalized, and the same team of doctors does not follow you from inside of the hospital to outside it. Large hospital systems have division of duties. Except for Bone Marrow Transplants, almost all treatments take place outside the hospital. Eventually the outpatient team will become your main point of contact.

Final treatment decisions often need to wait until the acute event like the pneumonia or gastric bleeding has resolved. The treatment will depend on many other factors that we will discuss further in Chapter 10 about Treatment Choices and in Chapter 14 concerning Goals of Treatment.

The Oncologist who will take over your care after you are discharged will become your main Oncologist. The Oncologist in the hospital is taking care of the immediate problem.

As in your financial life, you need someone who may help you with your long-term plans and someone else who takes care of your car loan. You need both, but they are different roles. Sometimes the people who help you overlap and interact. You can't get the car loan if you are not credit worthy. Similarly you need the hospital doctors to take care of you when you are admitted for your pneumonia and the Cancer Center doctors to take care of your long-term treatment

This scenario may repeat itself further along in your treatment if you need admission to the hospital. You will be seen by a different set of doctors inside and outside the hospital. Good communication between them is essential. If you are in the same hospital system using the same electronic records, your information will be visible to all the doctors. If you get treated in different hospital systems, the transfer of information is not as seamless and will need active management on your part. We will address this issue further in Chapter 9 on where you should be treated.

After John was discharged, he was seen in the Cancer Center, met with his team of Oncologists, and was given a treatment plan. From then on that team helped him manage his cancer treatment.

If you are hospitalized in a smaller center, hospital work and outpatient work is not quite so divided. You are more likely to be followed by the same doctors after you are discharged. The trend is towards division of duties, but it may not be quite as sharp. Large centers involve many different doctors.

Outside the hospital, as an outpatient...

If you were diagnosed outside the hospital, the next stage of your management is scheduled as an outpatient. You start with your Family (or Primary) doctor when you develop symptoms, and you have a scan that shows a tumor. The biopsy is done. If it shows cancer, your Family doctor sends you to the Cancer Center. The Cancer Center schedules additional consultations with the Medical and Radiation Oncologists. They will manage your care from here on.

Neal had his biopsy in the hospital, his condition stabilized, and he was discharged. Further consultations and testing then took place as an outpatient.

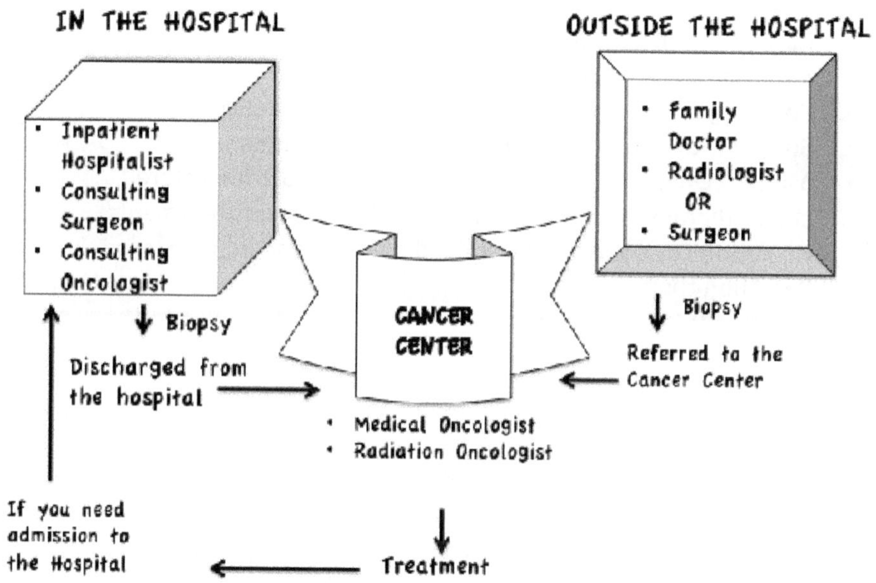

Figure 4.2

Who are the Doctors involved so far?

- **Primary Physician**: Family doctor who started the investigation.
- **Hospital team**: Internist and Specialists who treated you in the hospital.
- **Radiologist**: Read the scans.
- **Interventional Radiologist**: Did the biopsy.
- **Pathologist**: Examined the tissue and made the diagnosis.
- **Surgeon**: Operated for biopsy or to remove the tumor.
- **Medical Oncologist**: Determined need for and administered chemotherapy, hormone therapy or other Cancer treatments.
- **Radiation Oncologist**: Determined need for and administered Radiation therapy.

Action Plan: while you wait...

- If the cancer diagnosis is not certain, don't jump to a premature conclusion. Do focus on a healthy lifestyle.
- Quit smoking, if you smoke.
- Improve your diet.
- Exercise.

These lifestyle changes will help you whether your biopsy shows cancer or not.

Glossary

- Shadow/ lump/mass/tumor= Something that shouldn't be there.
- Biopsy= Sample of tissue taken from the suspicious site.
- Frozen Section=Quick look at the tissue from the site by the Pathologist during an operation.

5. What Does Your Pathology Report Mean?

So far we have been following the development of cancer cells, the biopsy, and the diagnosis of cancer. In this chapter we will start deciphering the biopsy results. When patients get a copy of their pathology report, the technical words are difficult to understand. In this chapter, we will review the meaning and significance of each component of the report.

Neal is discharged from the hospital after he has his biopsy. He has not coughed up any more blood, and it will take a few more days for the biopsy results. The next week, Neal and his wife, Mona, get a call from his family doctor. They meet with her to discuss the biopsy results. Their family doctor confirms that Neal has cancer and makes him an appointment with the Oncologist.

The pathology report is ready. The agonizing wait is finally over. The pathology report comes back and confirms cancer. When your family doctor shares this information, there are too many emotions flying through your brain to digest what it means. Your family asks for the pathology report so you can do your own internet search. The Oncologist's appointment is a few days away. How will you be able to figure out what this means without jumping to all the wrong conclusions?

What does the Pathology report mean?

Neal's report says in its conclusion:

"**Poorly differentiated, Grade 3 adenocarcinoma, with lymphovascular invasion and perineural invasion. Immunoperoxidase stains pending.** "

Does this mean that cancer cells are invading and running rampantly through your body? Is it invading all your blood vessels and nerves? Does grade 3 mean advanced cancer? How many grades are there?

These descriptive, technical words help identify and classify the cancer cell correctly. The medical definitions are different from colloquial English language definitions even if the words appear to be the same. Physicians need to use specific terms to make sure they are all referring to the same condition in a standardized way. This is important because it will help choose the right treatment.

If you were a machinist, for example, you would want the specs standardized so that you could order parts that fit correctly. Similarly, Oncologists and Pathologists use specific words for the descriptions.

Let us look at the components of the Pathology report.

The Pathologist will comment on:

1) **Organ of origin**, if possible. This may be easy if the biopsy is obviously from the organ of origin, or the Primary site, for example the breast, prostate, stomach, etc. If the biopsy is from a Secondary site, it may not always be possible to identify the organ of origin just from looking at the cells. Additional pathological clues like special immunoperoxidase stains for identifying specific proteins on the cell wall would help. And radiological clues with CT scans may be required to track down the original location of this cancer.

Why is this important? Cancers from different organs react differently to treatment and can have different treatments. For example, if the biopsy is from the bone, but the cell is identified to be similar to lung cancer cells, it will be called lung cancer. If the cell tests like a breast cancer cell, it will be called breast cancer. Breast and lung cancer treatments are different, and the treatment is directed against the kind of organ it came from, not the organ it landed in. They are both different from bone cancer treatments.

For example, if a basketball team were practicing on the gymnastics floor, the basketball players would be dribbling and doing layups. They would not be doing gymnastics routines. They would still be practicing basketball.

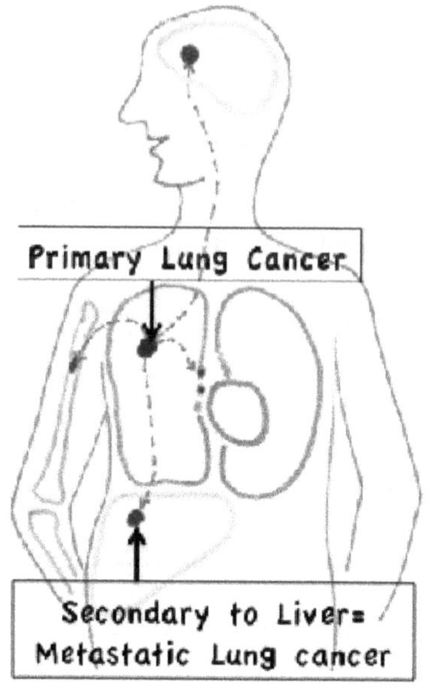

Figure 5.1

2) **The tissue of origin**: The different tissues in an organ develop different kinds of cancer. Cancer in the glands within the organ will give rise to an adenocarcinoma. Cancer in the surface lining in that same organ will develop into squamous cell carcinoma. Within the skin, different kinds of skin cancer can develop. For example, basal cell or squamous cell carcinoma or melanoma are all skin cancers, but they are treated differently.

Why is this Important? Choices of lung cancer adenocarcinoma chemotherapy drugs can be different from drugs for lung cancer squamous cell carcinoma or small cell lung cancer.

They took the biopsy from the liver; why are they calling it lung cancer?

Sometimes a biopsy is taken from the liver or the bone, but the pathology report calls it lung cancer. Why is that? Why is it not liver cancer, or bone cancer?

Each organ and associated cancer has a specific type of cell. The Pathologist looks at the actual cells from the biopsy, and in most situations, can tell which type of cancer you have no matter where in your body the biopsy was taken.

Treatment for lung adenocarcinoma will be different from colon adenocarcinoma, even if the disease is actually present in the liver. Bone cancer or liver cancer that started in the bone or the liver is treated differently from lung cancer which has spread to the bone or liver.

What makes an organ?

An organ consists of different kinds of tissues, glands and blood vessels with connective tissue holding it all together. It is surrounded by a capsule layer lining the outside of the organ. Cancer cells can develop from the same organ but from different tissues within the organ. E.g. Lung cancer can be either an adenocarcinoma or squamous cell carcinoma depending on which tissue became cancerous.

3) **Differentiation** describes how different the cancer cell looks from the normal cell. It ranges from well differentiated, where it more closely resembles the normal cell of origin, to poorly differentiated, where is it difficult to

recognize the tissue of origin.

I like to describe this as a room with walls, and the shape and furniture decides what kind of room it is. Is it a bedroom? It can be recognized as a bedroom if it has a bedroom set in it. Is it a dining room? Yes, if it has a dining room table. But what if there is no furniture? If there are just bare walls, and unidentifiable contents, it can be difficult to identify the room, and so it is with identifying the origin of the cell.

Why is this important? Undifferentiated cancer cells may behave more aggressively. They may be more resistant to standard treatment or tend to relapse faster. We may choose stronger treatment for more "undifferentiated" cancers.

The degree of differentiation will also be helpful in identifying the organ of origin. If the biopsy is from a secondary or metastatic site, and if the primary tumor cannot be identified, the cell gives us some clues about its origins. Sometimes the cell is too undifferentiated to be identified and treatment choices become more challenging. The cancer is now labeled a carcinoma of unknown primary.

4) **Grade** refers to the degree of disorganization inside the nucleus. The nucleus is the brain of the cell and contains the DNA, or genetic material of the cell. The normal DNA is arranged in chromosomes that have a regulated look. In cancer cells the DNA looks disorderly. A Grade 1 nucleus is less disorderly than a Grade 3 nucleus and, thus, Grade 1 is better behaving than Grade 3. In grade 1 disease, the nucleus looks like the gym during a physical education class. Even if the children are running around they are still following some instruction by the gym teacher. A grade 3 nucleus looks like recess on the playground where they are running helter-skelter.

The nucleus is graded from 1 to 3 or 4, depending on the specific cancer cell.

Why is Grade important? It is one more tool to try to anticipate future behavior of the cancer cells.

Note: Grade and stage should not be confused. We will discuss stage in Chapter 7. Stage refers to the map of the physical locations of the tumor; grade refers to characteristics of the nucleus of the cell. I have often had panicky patients who have read their pathology report, found Grade 3 disease, and thought they had the worse prognosis of Stage 3 disease. The Pathologist does not comment on the Stage from the initial biopsy.

Stage 1 Grade 3 disease is better than Stage 3 Grade 1 disease.

5) **Hormone Receptors**: Receptors are proteins on the cell surface that act like gateways or messengers to the inside of the cell (See Chapter 2). The hormone receptors that are commonly reported in breast cancer are receptors for estrogen and progesterone. Normally, hormones bind to their special receptors and send a signal to the inside of the normal cell to perform its specific function. The native, normal cell is driven by hormonal changes in the body. For example, fluctuations in estrogen levels are the reason why cysts in the breast can grow during certain periods in the menstrual cycle. When the cell turns cancerous, the receptors can be either lost or retained.

Why is this important? If the receptors are present, the cancer cell can continue to respond to changes of hormone levels. The cancer cell can be manipulated by using hormone-blocking therapy. When the receptors are lost, the behavior and growth of the cancer cell become independent of hormone levels. The cancer cell becomes "receptor negative" and does not respond to manipulation of its hormonal environment. The cancer cell is now functioning independently of hormone levels, and hormone manipulation does not work in receptor negative disease, For example, Estrogen Receptor (ER) and Progesterone Receptor (PR) negative breast cancer will not respond to estrogen blocking drugs.

Note: In Prostate Cancer, cells can initially respond to hormonal manipulation. They can become resistant as time goes by and stop responding to hormonal treatment.

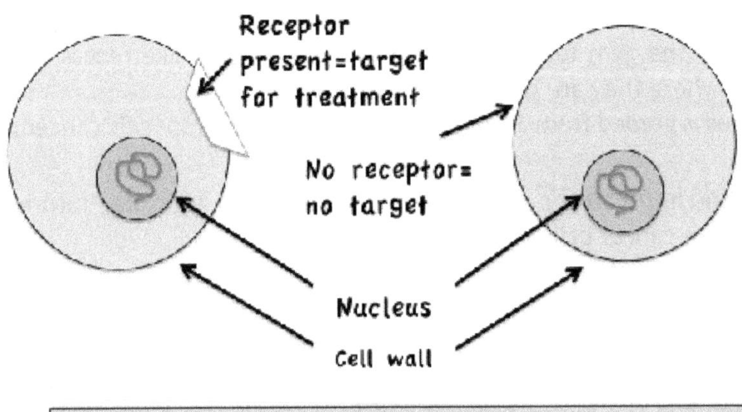

Figure 5.2

6) **Growth Factor Receptors**: A Growth Factor receptor is a special receptor on the cell surface that can be activated by circulating messenger chemicals. It then sends internal signals to the nucleus. Normally this regulates the normal growth and function of the cell. A mutation of this growth factor receptor can cause misfired growth signals and uncontrolled growth.

Why is this important? Presence or absence of a mutated EGFR (Epidermal Growth Factor Receptor) can help direct therapy with special designer drugs that target this receptor. This will be further addressed in the chapter on Treatment choices (Chapter 9).

"Behavior of the cancer cell"

What do we mean by the behavior of the cancer cell? If a cancer is low grade, responds well to treatment, has low risk of detaching from the primary site and causing secondary sites of disease, and has a low risk of relapse, it shows **good behavior**. A **badly behaving cell** tends to invade blood vessels or lymphatic vessels and cause secondary sites of disease. It does not respond well to standard treatment and has higher risk of early relapses. There is no direct measurement to predict behavior. It is a composite of many different factors. As more specialized testing is done on the cancer cell in the future, we will get better at predicting behavior.

Examples of Normal Hormone Function:

- Insulin regulates blood sugars.
- Thyroid hormone helps keep the engine of the body running.
- Pituitary hormones send messages to the testes and ovaries for puberty, sperm and egg production, menstrual cycles, pregnancy and lactation.
- The testes and ovaries produce testosterone, estrogen and progesterone to carry out reproductive functions.
- The adrenal glands produce steroid hormones and other messengers of the survival functions of the body.

All these functions are carried out by circulating hormones interacting with special receptors on the cell surface.

7) **Genetic mutations**: Mutations have become increasingly useful tools to detect additional targets of treatment. There are newer drugs that have been designed to work against these targets. These have produced breakthroughs in treatment for melanoma and kidney cancer that were mainly unresponsive to chemotherapy. In the future, the identification of genetic mutation targets may become more important than the tissue of origin.

8) **DNA signatures** yield a composite score which can predict a high or low risk of relapse and potential benefit with chemotherapy (e.g. Oncotype DX score which is used in breast cancer). A number of such scoring systems are being developed in different cancers to help predict risk of relapse and benefit from treatment.

Why is this important? If we can predict who will benefit from chemotherapy and who will not need it, or benefit from it, we can spare a number of people from undergoing unnecessary treatment. Chemotherapy is worth the side effects only if it will decrease the risk of recurrence. If there is a low risk of relapse, then additional chemotherapy may not be necessary and can be avoided in those patients. If there is a high risk of relapse, additional chemotherapy after surgery would be beneficial in reducing the risk and improving survival.

What are tumor markers?

Some cancers are associated with elevated blood levels of tumor markers. These are proteins that are shed into circulation by cancer cells as well as normal cells. They are not useful in early detection of cancer because they are not sensitive or specific enough, as we will discuss in the appendix on Screening. Their value lies in measuring response to treatment in advanced cancers once the cancer has been diagnosed and treated. If the number is elevated at the time of diagnosis, then watching the number go down is a reassurance that the cancer treatment is working. If the number is not elevated at the time of diagnosis, then for that person the tumor marker is not useful to measure disease response or disease progression. These blood tests are not part of the Pathology report but will be done as part of the initial diagnosis.

Examples of tumor markers that are used to monitor the response of the cancer to treatment are

- PSA- Prostate Cancer
- CA 19-9 - Pancreatic Cancer
- CEA-Colon Cancer, Lung Cancer

- CA 15-3, CA 29.29 – Breast Cancer
- CA 125- Ovarian Cancer

Why is my cancer called invasive?

Joan came in for her first consultation armed with her pathology report. She had had her routine mammogram, and a cluster of abnormal calcium deposits had been seen. She had been called back for a biopsy; a needle had been placed in the area, and a core sample was extracted for examination. No mass was felt, no enlarged lymph nodes were felt, but the biopsy confirmed *Invasive Ductal Carcinoma*. The word invasive sent chills down her spine, and by the time she had her first Oncology consultation, she was in a state of panic.

That is indeed a frightening word to see when you read your biopsy report. However it is not a description of how much cancer there is in your body. It does not mean that cancer cells are running amok and spreading to all your organs. It is a description of what the Pathologist sees under the microscope when he/she examines a sample of the tumor. There are specific demarcations in tissues which are natural boundaries like membranes surrounding glands or blood vessels. They mimic the walls around a gated community which separates the insiders from the outsiders. A breach in the wall only means that there is access. Similarly, when the tissue boundaries have been penetrated, or invaded, the description includes the word "invasive," This does give the cell the ability to spread, via the invaded blood or lymphatic vessels, but it does not mean it has actually spread. Whether it has spread or not will be determined by additional "staging" scans which determine the stage of the disease. We will address staging in Chapter 7.

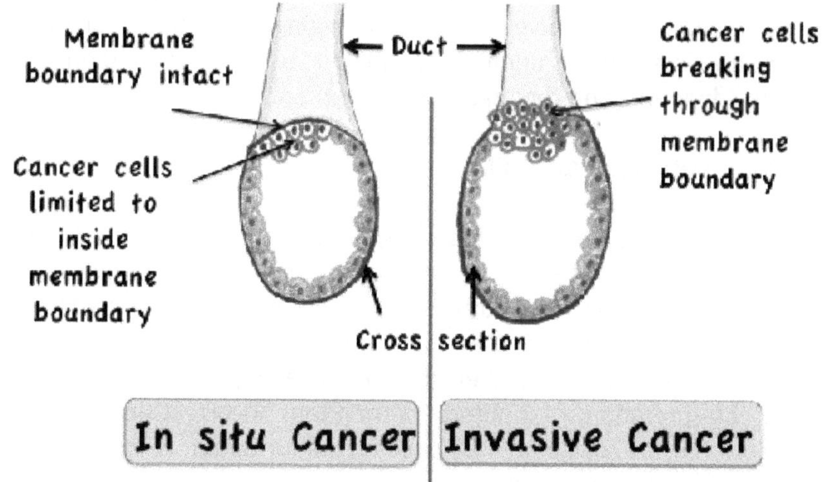

Figure 5.3

The word *invasive* differentiates the nature of the condition from *in situ*. In situ denotes that the natural barrier has not been invaded. In situ means "in place" and even if the changes in the cell can *look* cancerous, the condition is *not* cancer. It is still considered *pre-cancerous*. In situ disease does have a risk for becoming invasive disease in a small percentage of people, but it does not always need to be treated with the same aggressive measures as invasive disease.

In fact, there has been discussion afoot for many years to remove the word "cancer" from in situ disease. For example, seeing the word carcinoma in breast "DCIS" (or ductal carcinoma in situ) creates the same anxiety as invasive breast cancer and has led to an epidemic of aggressive over-treatment. In situ conditions should not carry fear of death; they only indicate a possibility of a recurrence which can turn invasive or cancerous. Predictive tools need to be developed as to which variety of DCIS carries a higher risk. There is a DNA score that has been developed for that purpose, but more work needs to be done to spare otherwise healthy people from overtreatment. This has been accomplished in cervical cancer where the management of invasive cervical cancer is different and more involved than that for in situ cervical cancer.

Let us revisit our example of a residential housing subdivision that we discussed in Chapter 2 on the development of the tumor. If there were a zoning violation, for example a house extension that was too close to the street, we would take care of the violator and monitor their behavior. We wouldn't raze the entire subdivision. That would be a disproportionate response and destroy an otherwise completely healthy neighborhood. Similarly, in situ pre-cancerous disease does not always need the same aggressive treatment as invasive cancer. In fact, it could lead to unwanted and unwarranted side-effects by destroying healthy tissue. Treating invasive disease, on the other hand, would require more aggressive measures like razing the entire subdivision.

What in situ disease does require is adequate local measures and ongoing monitoring, depending on the organ of involvement.

Correct Interpretation is Critical!

The importance of correctly interpreting the pathology report and putting it in the correct context cannot be overstated. I have had patients come in for their first consultation in a state of panic, because they had been doing research based on the report that they had received. Other patients have had wrong guidance given to them by well-meaning friends based on an incorrect interpretation of limited information. Incorrect interpretation causes more harm than good. Easy access to information is very valuable. Correct interpretation is even more so.

Neal's report: So what does Neal's Pathology report mean?

Neal has an adenocarcinoma, a cancer that is of glandular origin, as opposed to squamous, which comes from the lining. It is poorly differentiated, and they cannot yet identify it as a lung cancer, so they are doing additional "immunoperoxidase" stains to confirm the organ of origin. Circumstantially we know that he has a lung tumor, and the special stains may confirm whether the primary is in the lung or spread from elsewhere. Since it is poorly differentiated, this may not always be possible. The invasion of the blood and lymphatic vessels within the tumor site points to a worse behavior of the cancer cell, but the actual stage will be confirmed by scans.

Neal's next step is to see the Cancer Specialists. His consultations are scheduled for the next week.

Action Plan:

- Do not jump to conclusions. The initial biopsy report does not give the stage.
- Wait for your Oncology Consultation. Ask for an explanation.
- If you read your Pathology report, underline what you do not understand.
- Remember the technical words in the pathology report have different meanings than we understand in our common language.

Glossary

- Invasive= Penetrated natural boundary.
- In situ= Confined to defined lining layer.
- Grade= Description of nucleus.
- Differentiation= Description of cell.
- Receptor= Special gateway protein on cell membrane.
- Immunoperoxidase stains= Special dyes to help identify cells.

6. How to Prepare for Your Appointments

Neal and his wife, Mona, came for their first few appointments with their three grown children. Two of them lived in neighboring towns and one had flown in from another state. It was useful for them all to hear what the doctors had to say and ask their own questions. It was good for Neal and Mona to have a few more sets of ears and to have help in navigating this terrifying journey.

Not everyone has grown children or siblings close by, so use whatever resources you have. Your friends, neighbors, co-workers, or members of your temple or church may be happy to help, and don't be afraid to ask them. Your first few visits are overwhelming. You are facing new and unknown territory, and it is normal to be frightened. You are asked to make treatment choices that will affect your life. You don't understand how this could happen to you and you don't understand the words. If you don't understand what someone is saying, please don't be afraid to ask questions. This is your body and your life, and you are in a partnership with your health care team to get the best treatment available.

How do you prepare for your appointments?

Don't do it alone.

Gather your resources, your partner, children, siblings, friends, anyone who can help you digest this information. Take someone with you to help you listen and ask questions.

Take notes, use a recorder, and review what you don't understand. Your smart phone or tablet has a built in recording device. Don't hesitate to ask your doctor to explain something again. If you know the questions you want to ask in advance, write them down so you can be sure they are all addressed during your visit.

Keep your family informed, especially if you are close to them and they are involved in your care. If you have an extended family and friends and want to keep them all informed, consider setting up a blog or private social media page. If that is too much for you, designate someone who can pass on information to your family and friends. If you do this, you will not need to repeat what you have learned to everyone, you will be able to control the information flow, and it will help to reduce the number of phone calls, texts, and e-mails you receive.

Family conferences are useful for you, for your family and for your doctors. A family conference is an appointment which any of your family or friends that you would like to be involved may attend with you. The doctor can explain your disease to everyone, and people can ask questions. It is also useful for your doctor to get a sense of your support systems at home. If someone cannot be physically present, they can listen in by speakerphone. Family conferences can be arranged initially when you are diagnosed and repeated at future critical decision points.

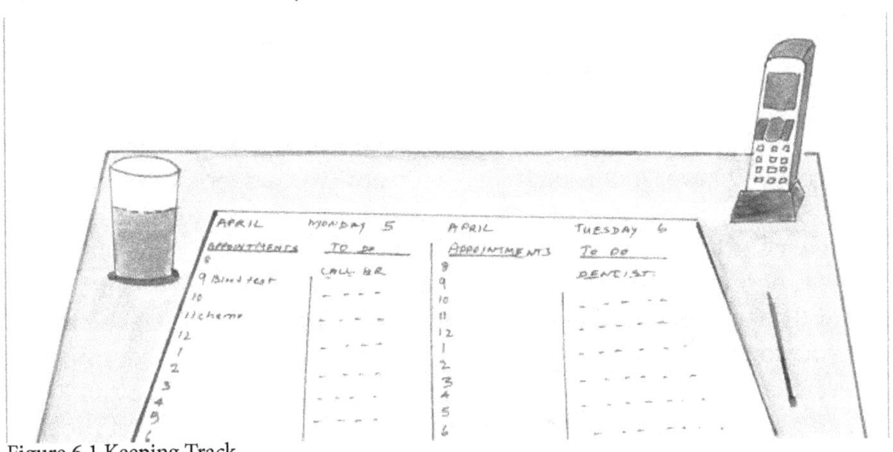

Figure 6.1 Keeping Track

Keep track

As the initial consultation leads to other appointments and visits, keeping a calendar becomes necessary.

An Agenda book/ Diary/ Calendar keeps track of

- Future appointments--both treatment visits and doctor visits
- Test results
- List of medications which will need to be kept current
- Instructions regarding side effects
- Instructions regarding nutrition/ fluid intake
- Questions to ask at your next visit
- Contact numbers for your treating physicians.

Electronic calendars on your phone are convenient for you to keep track of your appointments. If different people are going to attend different appointments, however, a paper agenda book or diary can make it easier for them to take notes which they can then share and pass on to the next person who comes with you. The diary or agenda book can function like a baton in a relay. This helps keep the continuity of your instructions in one place.

After your initial consultation, you will have regular visits with your Oncology team both during and after your treatments. Remember to write down your concerns and questions. Refer to your list at the end of your visit to make sure your questions have all been answered.

Managing your other Medical problems:

You will still have to manage other medical conditions that are unrelated to your cancer--high blood pressure, diabetes, heart disease, or ordinary infections.

If you also see a Cardiologist or Endocrinologist in addition to your Primary doctor, you will need to continue to visit them. Most Oncologists will not manage your heart condition or your diabetes. They will prefer that you continue your care with the other specialists.

It is important that all your doctors communicate with each other. If they have electronic medical records and are on the same computer system, they can view each other's notes. If, however, your Primary physician is in one hospital system, your Cardiologist in another, and your Orthopedic doctor in a third, they cannot easily share your information. Electronic communication has to be encrypted for security reasons, and there is no "cross talk" between systems. It then becomes even more important for you to keep good records yourself.

Neal has started keeping an agenda book. He has created sections for his appointments, his questions for visits, and his list of medicines. He adds the names and numbers of his doctors and pharmacy. You will find additional suggestions for record keeping in the appendix in the section on Checklists. Neal's son has set up a private social media page so the family can keep each other informed.

Action Plan

- Gather your resources: List family, friends, neighbors, and co-workers who want to help.
- Be organized: Keep your records and an agenda book.
- Follow instructions.
- Write down your questions.
- Turn on your answering machine or voicemail.
- Turn off call blocking for unknown numbers. Your doctors' offices will be calling you. They need to be able to reach you.

7. What Is Staging?

Neal and Mona waited a week for the biopsy report and another four days for their first oncology consultation. At this point they have pored over his pathology report (see Chapter 5) and their children have scoured the internet for answers. They are eager to start treatment, but they learn that the doctors have not finished gathering all the necessary information. We will need to Stage the cancer. This step is critical to determine the treatment plan.

What is staging?

Staging is a standardized way of measuring all the places the disease is located. To stage your cancer, the doctors map all locations in your body where the disease is present. Cancer commonly starts in one organ, the primary site, and spreads to other areas, the metastatic or secondary sites. These areas are detected either during surgery or with a variety of special scans.

Stages start from early, or Stage 1, to the late, Stage 4. Three components are involved in staging the cancer.

T: Tumor size ranges from T1 to T4, with T1 being the smallest.

N: indicates involvement of lymph nodes and ranges from N0-N3. N0 indicates that no lymph nodes have been invaded by cancer cells. N1 indicates that very few lymph nodes have been affected; N2 and N3 indicate an increasing number of affected lymph nodes.

M: indicates distant or metastatic spread. M 0 indicates no distant disease, and M 1 indicates it is present. If distant disease is present, the stage automatically jumps to Stage 4 no matter how small the primary tumor or how small the distant disease.

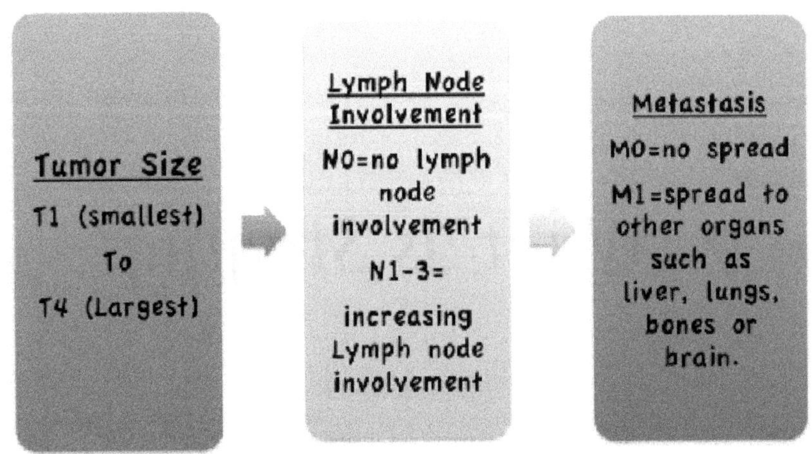

Stage is a combination of T, N and M,

for example:

T1N0M0=Stage 1 and T1N1M1=Stage 4

Figure 7.1 Staging of Cancer

The Stage is a final composite of the extent of T, N, M classification. (See Figure 7.1) For example, T1N0M0 describes a Stage 1 disease; T1N1 M1 describes Stage 4 disease. Any M1 becomes Stage 4. Cancers of different primary origins have different criteria for determining the T and the N portions depending on the local anatomy. For example, breast tumors are measured according to their size, or rectal tumors are categorized according to their depth of penetration. In different organs, different factors contribute to the risk of spread.

Each Cancer has its own rules of measurement. For Example, in Breast Cancer:

T1 mi= 0-1 mm	N0 = no nodal involvement.
T1a=1-5 mm	N1 = level 1 or 2 axillary nodes involved, not fixed.
T1b=5-10 mm	N2 = fixed or matted axillary lymph nodes.
T1c=11-20 mm	N3 = lymph nodes in neck, collarbone or inframammary regions.
T2 to T4=increasing size of tumor.	

Why is Staging so important?

Treatment for Stage 1 disease is very different from treatment for Stage 4 disease. In each kind of cancer, fixed criteria measure the primary tumor size, the surrounding lymph nodes, and the distant sites.

"Why did we have to wait to start the staging scans? Aren't we losing time?"

When planning a trip, in order to reach your destination, you need to correctly confirm your position on the map. In order to complete staging, cancer has to be confirmed; you cannot start the scans unless the biopsy confirms cancer. Different kinds of scans may be needed for different kinds of cancers, or, if the biopsy report comes back normal or benign, additional scans are not necessary. Some scans take place during the diagnostic investigation. After cancer is confirmed, a series of scans is scheduled.

Scans are non-invasive tests that look at the inside of the body. They often require the injection of intravenous dye, or you may need to drink an opaque liquid. The dye helps to distinguish the tumor from normal tissue and to properly read the images.

Which scans may be done?

An **Ultrasound** is a non-invasive way of looking inside your body. The machine has a handle that is moved over your skin, outside your body. It sends ultrasound waves (sound waves whose pitch is higher than the human ear can detect) into the body, and the different structures reflect the sound waves back, making a picture. It is like the sonic images submarines use to "look" at their surroundings. Ultrasound technology also looks for cysts or fluid collections, blood flow through the heart, or blocked ducts in the gall bladder or kidney. When used with special internal probes for the food pipe (esophagus) or rectum, it can reveal how deep the tumor has penetrated. This helps to plan possible surgery.

A **CAT or CT scan (Computer Aided Tomography)** machine is like a large doughnut, and the patient lies on a platform that travels through it. The machine sends X-rays across your body as you pass through it. The cross-sectional X rays produce pictures that reflect the insides of your body. Better pictures are obtained when dye is injected and/or swallowed to better outline the target organs. The injected dye has the potential to cause an allergic reaction, however, and it needs to be used with caution in people whose kidneys do not function well. Therefore, depending on the target, CT scans are sometimes done without injecting the dye.

An MRI is a Magnetic Resonance Imaging scan. This machine looks similar to the CT Scanner above, but it uses electro-magnetic waves generated by large magnets in a closed space. The magnetic field changes the alignment of the protons in the cells. The waves bounce off the different tissues of the body with different intensity producing images of the internal tissue. The accuracy of the picture is improved by injecting a special dye which spreads through the tissue and helps with the magnetic alignment of the protons in the tissue.

The MRI scan can take 30-60 minutes to complete. The part of the body being scanned is positioned inside the scanner portion of the machine, and the person has to lie perfectly still on the table. The magnet is loud, and the confinement can be difficult for people with claustrophobia. Some people may need to take a small dose of anti-anxiety medicine before the procedure. Others may use headphones with music if available at the facility.

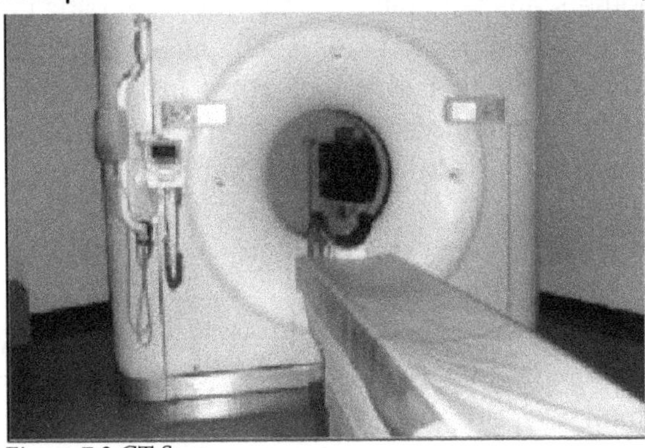

Figure 7.2 CT Scan

Why perform a CT scan instead of an MRI (or vice versa)? CT scans are quick and easier for patients with claustrophobia. They give better pictures of bony structures and solid organs. CT scans do involve exposure to radiation because they use X rays. MRIs produce better images for soft tissues like nerves, ligaments, the brain, and the spinal cord, but they take longer and the patient has to lie still for a long time. MRIs use magnetic waves, not radiation. Because of the use of magnets, however, people who have certain kinds of metal (for example artificial valves, stents, or prosthetics) in their body cannot have an MRI. Each scan has its uses, benefits, and drawbacks.

A **bone scan** looks for hot spots (or areas of increased activity) in the bones. A radioactive dye is injected into the blood stream via an IV. The dye is absorbed by the bone cells. A few hours later the scanner picks up the radioactivity and produces an image. The presence of cancer in the bones has a characteristic appearance producing "hot spots" which take up more dye than normal areas. This level of radioactivity is very safe and differs from radiation treatment. Other processes in the bones also produce an abnormal scan, for example a healing fracture or arthritis. The picture is different, and the clinical situation helps in making the diagnosis.

A bone scan differs from a bone density test which does not detect the presence or absence of cancer. The bone density scan is done only to look for osteoporosis. It does not involve the injection of radioactive dye. The two tests are not interchangeable.

A **PET scan** looks for evidence of activity in an abnormal area, not just the structure. Whereas CAT scans and MRIs can only look for the physical evidence of tumors, PET scans detect function to differentiate live cells from scar tissue.

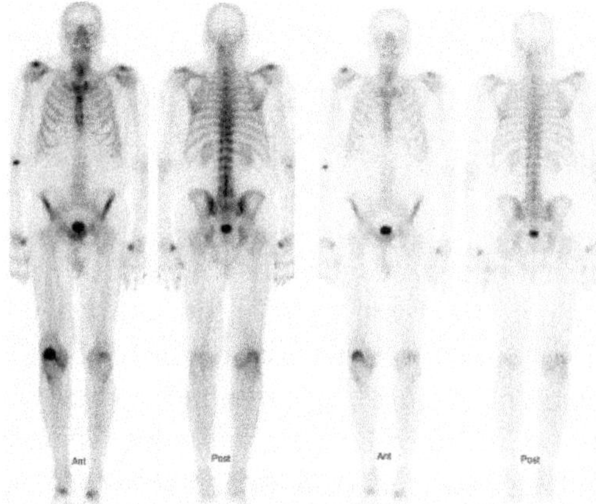

Figure 7.3 Bone Scan Images

A solution of a radioactive isotope, like radio-labeled glucose (or another radioactive compound in a safe and standardized dose) is injected into the blood stream. The glucose is actively taken up by areas of increased activity (cancer cells, infections, healing tissue after an operation, pneumonia). Scar tissue does not take up much glucose, so this test can differentiate between an old scar and active cancer. Scars are commonly present and show up as shadows on the CT scan. Scars (internal and external) can be a residual effect of previous injury and not be cancer, but they can be difficult to tell apart in a CT scan. A PET scan is also useful to determine if the disease has been eradicated or is or is not responding to therapy.

Different instructions for each scan will be given to you before you go for the test.

Is the disease localized, or has it spread?

Scans help to determine the extent of disease. Is the cancer limited to the primary organ, like the breast, lung, or colon, or has it spread to secondary organs like the liver, lungs, bones, or brain?

The stage of the disease will ultimately be decided by a combination of surgical findings, final pathology reports, and the staging scans. If the tumor is removed, the Pathologist can measure the actual tumor size, involvement of any lymph nodes in the sample, and any evidence of spread in the body cavity. If the tumor is treated without surgery, the stage is determined by scans.

Staging a tumor:

1) **Determines treatment**: What works for Stage 3 may be overkill for Stage 1. Surgical treatment that may be appropriate for Stage 1 will not be appropriate for Stage 4. Overtreatment exposes you to side effects, some of which can be worse than the cancer.

2) **Helps with prognosis**: It will give an approximate idea of what the expectation of survival can be. This will be different with each stage. Stage 1 disease has a better chance of cure than Stage 3.

Neal's next step:

Neal and Mona's visit ends with scheduling a Brain MRI and a PET scan to complete the staging. Neal will have a consultation with a Radiation Oncologist and a Chest Surgeon as part of a multidisciplinary evaluation. In the next chapter we will discuss the consultation process further. Neal's case will be presented in a Tumor Board Conference which will include the Pathologist and Radiologist. His biopsy slides and scans will be reviewed, and a treatment plan appropriate to his stage will be recommended.

Action Plan

- Ask to record the consultation so you can go back and listen to the explanation.
- If a vital member of your family is not able to attend, ask if they can listen in on a speaker-phone connection in the room.
- Start keeping a calendar/diary to keep track of appointments, your questions, the answers and instructions.
- Designate one person as a note taker and contact person.
- Update your contact information at the doctor's office.
- Make sure your voice mail or answering machine is activated. Check your messages.

Glossary

- Staging= Determining extent of disease and mapping all the locations of the disease.
- Primary Site= Where the disease starts.
- Secondary or Metastatic site= Place where the disease spreads.
- Lymph node= Normal collection of cells along the lymphatic circulation that filter the lymph fluid and process immunity.

"When you have exhausted all possibilities, remember this. You haven't."

Thomas Edison
Inventor

Section C

Treatment:
How, Where, What, Why?

8. How Are Treatment Decisions Made?

Neal starts his treatment planning. After Neal and Mona have their first consultation with the Oncologist, Neal completes his staging scans. Then they return to the Oncologist to discuss treatment. They are going to meet with the Medical Oncologist, the Radiation Oncologist, and the Thoracic Surgeon who will review the scans and pathology, determine the stage, and make a recommendation for treatment.

You will get a lot of information in these consultations. You and your doctors will be making some important decisions. It is usually a good idea to bring along a family member or trusted friend as a second pair of ears and to take notes during these discussions about scans, test results, and treatment options.

Treatment decisions: How are these decisions made?

When a biopsy confirms cancer, an Oncologist, or cancer specialist, is consulted. There are two kinds of Oncologists: a Radiation Oncologist who specializes in radiation therapy and a Medical Oncologist who oversees chemotherapy and coordinates the care. Surgeons can specialize in cancer surgery especially if they are connected to a University hospital. In the local or community hospitals, surgery is often performed by General Surgeons who have a special interest or training in cancer surgery.

The three specialists from Surgery, Radiation, and Medical Oncology will confer about what treatment would be best for each individual patient. In the past the sequence of treatment was usually surgery followed by chemotherapy, radiation therapy, both, or nothing. In the last 25 years different sequences or combinations of treatment have shown improved outcomes. It is important to get the sequence correct in the initial review and treatment planning. Some cancers are treated with surgery first, and some benefit from pre-surgical treatment with radiation and chemotherapy which may enable a better, curative operation. Some cancers do not require any surgery and can be effectively treated with radiation and/or chemotherapy. The doctors' recommendation will depend on the disease and the stage, and it will be tailored to the patient's needs. They will make their recommendations based on current standard of care and national guidelines. They will also assess whether the patient needs to be referred to a specialty center or if participating in a clinical trial would be helpful. (We will discuss the functional assessment or performance status in Chapter 9.)

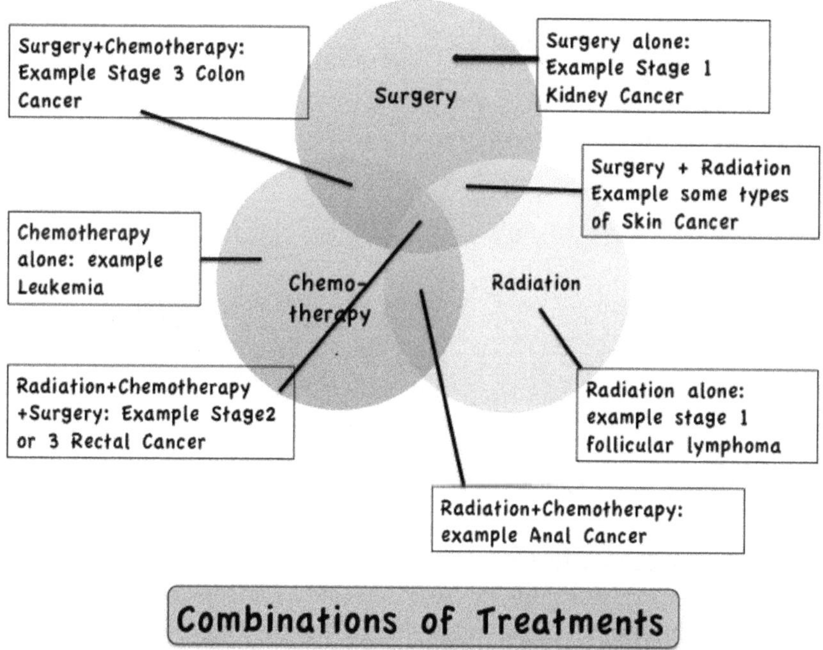

Figure 8.1

Consultation Settings:

Cancer treatment requires a coordinated treatment plan that can involve surgery, radiation, and chemotherapy. These consultations, reviews, and recommendations can take place in a variety of settings: multidisciplinary clinics, disease centers, individual consultations, or discussions at tumor boards.

What is a Multidisciplinary Clinic?

At a multidisciplinary clinic, a patient meets with all the specialists in one session. They will review the biopsy findings with the Pathologist and the radiological studies (like CT scans, MRIs, mammograms) with the Radiologist, have a conference, and recommend a course of action. If you are seeing these doctors for a second opinion, they will send their recommendation to the team that is treating you. If they are your treating team, they will arrange for the next step in the process.

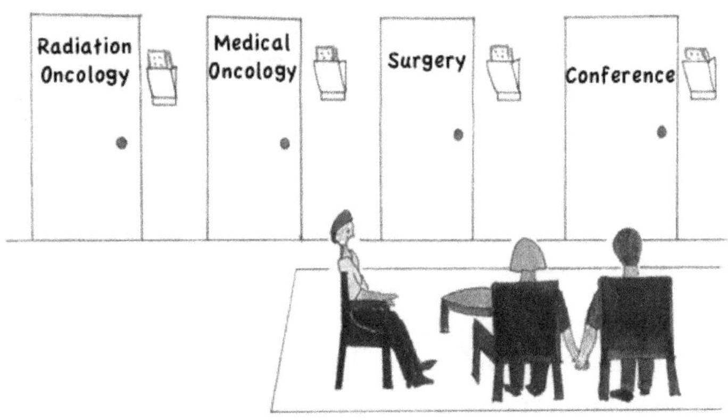

Multi Disciplinary Clinic

Figure 8.2

What are Disease Centers?

At major academic hospitals or large specialty Cancer Centers, clinics are organized into individual disease centers (for example a Breast Cancer Center or a Gastro-Intestinal Cancer Center).

The Oncologists at the disease centers only see patients with a specific cancer on their designated days at the center. They are also focused on clinical research. This setting is useful when you have a cancer that is not commonly seen in your local community.

What is a Tumor Board?

In some settings the review of your information takes place in a conference called a tumor board. This takes place without the patient physically present because the cases of many different patients are being discussed one after another, and many different team members are present. Patient confidentiality would be difficult to preserve if all those patients were in the room. At the

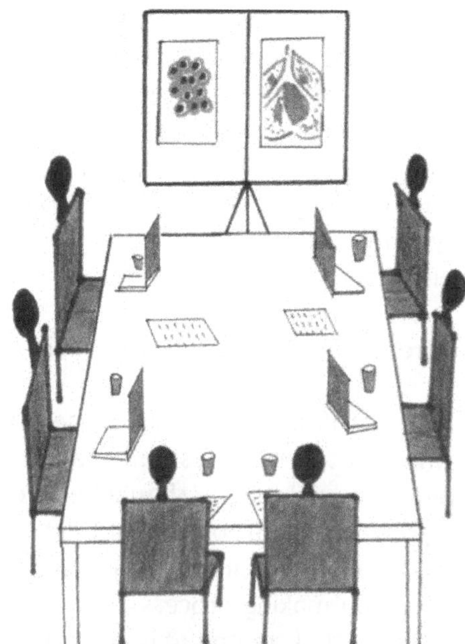

Figure 8.3 Tumor Board Meeting

tumor Board, after the lead physician talks about the case, the Pathologist reviews the slides, and the Radiologist reviews the scans, the group discusses the case and gives a recommendation for treatment that is sent to the referring physicians. The patient learns about the recommendations when he meets to consult with the specialists.

What if there is no Multidisciplinary Clinic in your area?

When there is no designated multidisciplinary clinic, the patient goes to the different consultant's offices separately and at different times. The doctors then confer and present a treatment plan to the patient. Inter-physician discussion takes place even without a formal multidisciplinary clinic. Tumor Boards discuss challenging cases, and visiting experts may participate in these discussions. Doctors may call or e-mail an expert elsewhere for advice. In these days of electronic communication, your physical location does not limit the ability of your doctors to communicate with each other.

Is a Multidisciplinary clinic visit essential?

In straightforward situations, a formal multidisciplinary clinic visit is not essential. In towns without large Cancer Centers it is difficult for specialists to coordinate a separate, dedicated time every week for individual diseases like lung cancer, breast cancer, or colon cancer. Doctors see patients any day of the week they are diagnosed. Even if a formal multidisciplinary clinic visit is not essential, it is necessary for the patient to consult with all the specialists.

What is essential is that all the consultants talk to each other, they review the pathology and x-rays findings, present all the options to you, explain their recommendations, and coordinate a plan of care.

Patient Navigator: Some facilities provide a patient navigator. This is often a nurse who will help you make these appointments and move the process along in a timely fashion.

National Standardized Treatment Guidelines: " Standard of care" is standard.

Treatment plans are standardized for each disease and stage. National cancer treatment organizations and professional cancer societies develop guidelines that are widely followed, so you should be able to be treated in a similar standardized way wherever you go for treatment. Recommendations change as new studies provide new information, but these changes are incorporated into the decision-making process. Each Cancer Center has its own internal reviews to insure that treatment is being delivered according to usual guidelines.

There are two main categories of Cancer Centers.

Referral Centers or Specialty Centers are located at University Hospital Centers. There the oncologist usually treats only one kind of cancer and is often involved in a research program related to that cancer.

Community hospitals are local hospitals which often have a Cancer Center. Oncologists here are not dedicated to a single cancer type; they treat all varieties.

When should I go to a University Cancer Center?

It is very useful to go to a University Cancer Center when you have a less common kind of cancer. In that situation the local hospital Cancer Center may not have the necessary familiarity with treatment options, treatment may not be standardized, and experimental treatment may be necessary which is only available at major Cancer Centers. Often your initial consultation with your local oncologists will determine the necessity of making the trip.

***

I got a call from a friend whose husband had just been diagnosed with cancer of the esophagus, or food pipe. She was searching the web for the "best place" to be treated, and she was thinking of travelling 2000 miles to be seen there. My friends lived in Chicago, Illinois, and had access to excellent care locally. My friend needed reassurance that her husband would get the state of the art treatment close to home, and it turned out they were very happy with that choice. Travelling to the "best" Cancer Center, which may not be close by, can be a hardship. Going through treatment far away from home is logistically difficult and expensive, and it may not be necessary.

***

Many years ago, a friend who lived overseas contacted me for advice. She was young and had just received a diagnosis of "triple negative breast cancer." This is a more aggressive variety of breast cancer. It had been caught early, in Stage 1, but the nature of the cell, the size of the primary tumor, and her premenopausal status put her at an increased risk for a recurrence. A Radiation Oncologist, not a Medical Oncologist, saw her. He was going to treat her with radiation, but he determined that she did not need chemotherapy and could be treated with a lumpectomy and radiation alone. He then proposed putting her on Tamoxifen, a pill that blocks the Estrogen receptor.

Was that an appropriate treatment? Since she was "receptor negative," she could not benefit from Tamoxifen, which is an estrogen receptor blocker. Did she need chemotherapy in addition to surgery and radiation therapy? I reviewed her reports and sent her the information about postoperative chemotherapy in addition to radiation therapy. She then went to the University Center, and they did proceed with chemotherapy, which would be the standard recommendation. If the Medical Oncologist had seen her in addition to the Radiation Oncologist, the treatment could easily have been done at her local Cancer Center, but the all the necessary specialists had not seen her.

***

Unfortunately, as a patient, it is hard for you to know which specialist is correct. So, while it is not necessary to go to a multidisciplinary clinic or a University Hospital for treatment, it is a useful resource as a second opinion.

So, should I get a second opinion?

Yes, if you have any concerns about what to do. You should not hesitate to seek a second opinion. It is reassuring to both the patient and the physician when there is agreement about the treatment plan. The consensus also builds your confidence in your team. When I was working in the community setting, and my patients went to get a second opinion, almost all of them returned to get their treatment from me. The patients who stayed at the referral center usually stayed because it was an unusual cancer or there were family or logistical reasons for the switch. In the end, we all want what is best for the patient.

Second opinions are very useful to:
a) Review the pathology.
b) Review treatment options.
c) Reassure you that the recommendations are appropriate.
d) Consider clinical trials.

Cancer Centers that provide second opinions do not require that you be treated at their center. You can return to your primary center for treatment. If the disease is not common, the Oncologists at the two centers can work collaboratively as well. Oncologists in the community hospitals often reach out to their academic colleagues at referral centers for difficult cases.

Neal and Mona decided to explore his options further. They wanted to make sure that he was going to receive the current state-of-the-art treatment. They also wanted to see if there were any clinical trials that would be preferred in his situation. They asked for a referral to the University Cancer Center.

Treatment Guideline Sources

- www.nccn.org
- www.cancer.gov
- http://www.instituteforquality.org/practice-guidelines

Action Plan

- Ask questions about Stage and Prognosis: What is my Stage? What is the outcome with treatment? What is the outcome without treatment?
- Ask about treatment options: Do I need surgery/ chemotherapy/ radiation therapy? What is best for my Stage? Can I tolerate it?
- Should I enroll in a clinical trial?
- Ask about a second opinion: Ask whom your doctor recommends?
- Ask if there is a Patient Navigator who can help you arrange the consultations.

Glossary

- **Tumor Board Conference**= Conference involving different specialists who review scans and pathology without the patient present.
- **Multidisciplinary Clinic**= Patient is seen by different cancer specialists (Medical and Radiation Oncology and Surgery) in one setting.

9. Where Should I Be Treated?

Neal was seen by the specialists at the University cancer center. Neal and Mona now face another major question: Where should Neal be treated? Neal could stay with his current team of doctors at his local hospital. He has known his Primary Care doctor for many years and trusts her. He lives close to the local hospital, and they do have a cancer center. If he went to the major cancer center at the University, he would have to fight rush hour traffic going into the city and pay for parking. His friends and family are pulling him in different directions.

Should you go to a University Cancer Center?

The major (or referral) cancer centers are located at a University and sometimes at specialty cancer centers, for example the Dana Farber Cancer Center in Boston, MA, the MD Anderson Cancer Center in Houston, TX, the Memorial Sloan Kettering Cancer Center in New York, NY, or the National Cancer Institute near Washington, D.C. Patients seek them out because they have read that they are the best in the country. Other patients are referred to the centers because their uncommon cancers need experimental treatment or, having received their initial treatment locally, the cancer has returned, and they are now seeking experimental treatment.

The pros:

At the tertiary, or referral centers, someone who is a specialist in the kind of cancer you have sees you. This may be important particularly if you have an uncommon cancer. You may benefit from enrolling in a clinical trial. You may have access to experimental drugs. More treatment is usually available at these centers when the previous one has failed. Most of these centers have nurses, social workers, and other care providers who work with specific "disease teams."

If your cancer is being treated with a standard protocol, however, there is no reason not to get treatment and care at your local hospital.

The cons:

The University or Specialty center is usually far from home. You have to travel and stay in hotels while you get your treatments. Your doctor is involved in research and can be away at meetings. You may have to see other people in the clinic who you have not met before--covering MDs, Nurse Practitioners, and Physician Assistants. If the cancer continues to grow, there is always another treatment option and another clinical trial or one more experimental drug. It is difficult to know when to stop trying more treatment. More treatment may not be the right thing to do.

Should you continue your care locally?

Local community hospitals do have cancer specialists who deliver chemotherapy and radiation therapy. community cancer centers must comply with and pass regulatory inspections. The oncologists are experienced and are usually board certified. They have trained at the University centers and keep up with the advances in treatments. If you have a cancer whose treatment is standard, you will be able to receive treatment locally without any difficulty. If you have an uncommon cancer, however, your local oncologists may suggest you receive treatment at the referral center.

The pros:

You are close to home and don't have to travel when you are not feeling well. You know the local hospital, your specialists are accessible, they know each other, and you can easily communicate with your Primary physician. Your support systems are in place. Remember, when you are treated at the local hospital, your oncologists did their training at a University cancer center.

The cons:

Clinical trials may not be available, and experimental drugs are not available. You may wonder whether you are getting the state of the art treatment.

Common versus uncommon conditions

If you have an uncommon disease, it makes sense to be seen by a specialist for that particular disease. If you have a common cancer, it's probably better to get a second opinion and return home for treatment. It's closer, and you will see your own oncologist every time you need to be seen.

How do I know if I am getting good quality care?

ACOS Certification of Cancer Centers

In the United States all cancer centers, whether in a referral center, at the University, or in the community, can be certified by the American College of Surgeons, or ACOS. The ACOS examines the policies and procedures of each Center every two to three years to insure safety and quality control. Unless deficiencies are corrected, the center does not get ACOS certification.

QOPI (Quality Oncology Practice Initiatives) Certification of Cancer Centers

In the USA cancer centers can be QOPI certified by The American Society of Clinical Oncology. The certification verifies their adherence to standard practice guidelines and their use of quality control measures. As a result you can rely on cancer care in any geographical area of the United States complying with standards. Other countries are also taking steps to ensure adherence to guidelines.

Can I get my treatment at a University Cancer Center and go to my local Cancer Center or my local ER if I am not feeling well?

You can do that. In some areas there is no cancer center at the local hospital. There is no choice but to go to the University hospital. Patients travel for the cancer treatments, and when they run into emergencies, their local family doctor sees them. Other times, patients are being treated at the University center because they choose to do so, or they are on an experimental treatment.

Why it is important to keep track of your treatment information...

In an emergency visit to a hospital that is not your cancer hospital, doctors may not get your relevant information quickly. If you arrive at the local emergency room with a fever during the midpoint of your chemotherapy cycle, doctors will need to know if you have already received an injection to boost your white cell count. If they cannot find that information, you may receive unnecessary treatment if your white cell count is low, or treatment may be delayed while they search for that information. Two different hospital system's medical records are not transparent to each other. During nights and weekends there is very limited information available to the non-treating center. So, if you have a choice and it is geographically possible, try to go to the same hospital system where you are receiving your cancer treatments so doctors can look at your treatment record and take the appropriate action.

What if you must go to different hospital systems for your care?

Keep your own meticulous records and take them with you to the hospital.

- Name and stage of your cancer.
- Chemotherapy drugs you are receiving and the number of treatments you have received.
- Date of your last treatment and any additional post treatment injections.
- Names of all prescription and non-prescription medicines you are taking.
- Dates and reasons for your hospitalizations.
- Dates and results of your last scans.
- Dates and results of your last blood work.
- Name and number of your treating Oncologist.

This information will help any team treat you in an emergency. You will find charts you can use in the Appendix.

How do I decide where to receive treatment?

The decision may depend on where you live. If you live in an urban area, it may be easy to seek a University-based academic cancer center without too much travel. If you live in a smaller town or rural area, doctors with the necessary expertise may not be readily available. You may need to travel for a second opinion or even stay there for treatment. Ideally your local oncologist and referral care consultant can confer, and you can be treated locally.

In the end, you have to find your comfort zone. You may choose to go to a University cancer center for a second opinion and return to your local cancer center for your treatment, or you could choose to stay at the University cancer center. You may have confidence in your local doctors and not go anywhere else at all.

Neal asked his primary doctor what she would do. She agreed with getting a second opinion at the University center and having another team review his pathology slides, confirm the diagnosis, and review his case to see if there were any additional treatment options. Since she had full confidence in his local team, she recommended staying close to home if the treatment were the same.

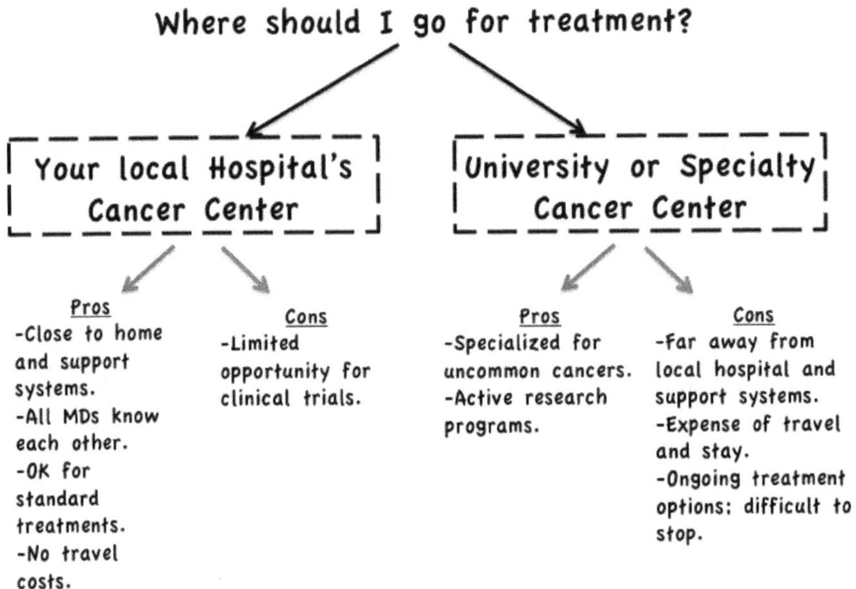

Figure 9.1

Points to consider when deciding where to be treated:

- Where do you live? Are you far from an academic cancer hospital?
- Do you have board certified oncologists at your local hospital?
- Is your cancer common or uncommon?
- What are your resources for travel?

Who are your doctors at this point?

- Primary care doctor.
- Surgeon managing any surgical issues.
- Local oncologist at the community cancer center.
- Specialty oncologist at the University.
- Other specialists you may need for kidney or heart disease or diabetes.

Action Plan:

- Ask your local oncologist if they work with a tertiary care center.
- Verify that your local cancer center is ACOS or QOPI certified.
- Verify that your local oncologists are board certified.
- Seek a second opinion.
- Weigh the pros and cons of where you are treated.
- Find your own comfort zone.

10. What Are the Treatment Choices?

Neal and Mona have come to their oncologist visit with many questions about his treatment plan. They had heard on the evening news about a new treatment that was very promising for lung cancer. Could they use that for Neal?

In the past patients used to go through surgery first and chemotherapy or radiation therapy afterwards. Today surgery is not necessarily the first or the only approach to treatment, and treatment has become a combination of many options. Surgery, chemotherapy, and radiation therapy (with an assist from hormone therapy) are still currently the mainstays of curative treatment, and we will discuss them in detail in Chapters 11-13. Several newer treatments have added promise in recurrent or advanced disease where curative options are otherwise limited. We will discuss them in this chapter.

The Main Categories of Treatment:

1) Surgery is used for several purposes:

a) **Diagnosis and biopsy**: When tissue cannot be obtained by a less invasive procedure, sometimes a limited surgery may be necessary. A small piece of the tumor is removed for analysis. Further treatment will be decided after the biopsy results are obtained. Curative surgery can only be done after the diagnosis because additional steps are needed to determine whether curative surgery can be performed.

b) **Curative surgery** intends to remove all evidence of cancer, and it is usually performed when preoperative testing shows the tumor is limited in extent. Here the entirety of the tumor is removed along with local lymph nodes and sometimes the surrounding organs. While this may be the intent at the outset of the surgery, whether that is feasible will depend on what the surgeon finds during the operation. There may be more disease than was visible on scans, or the tumor may be stuck to vital structures and unable to be safely and entirely removed.

In general a curative operation cleanly removes the tumor and the required surrounding tissues. Adequate tissue around the tumor site (**the margin**) needs to be cancer free. If the margins are not cancer free, the cancer cells left behind will grow back to make more tumors. Sometimes an operation needs to be repeated to clean the margins. This is mainly possible for cancers on the surface of the body, like breast or skin cancers. Cancers of internal organs are usually not amenable to repeat attempts at surgery because the body cavity may already be compromised by cancer cells and more surgery will not make it cancer free. If the cancer cannot be entirely removed, most often the operation is called off, and the patient proceeds with other management.

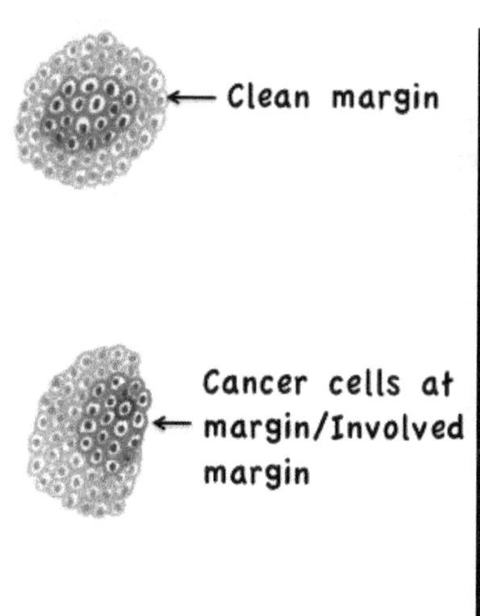

What is a margin?

A margin is the extent of cancer -free tissue that surrounds the tumor when it is surgically removed. A clean margin indicates that the tumor was cleanly removed. A close margin or an involved margin indicates that cancer cells are present at or near the edge of the removed tumor, and cancer cells may be left behind after the surgery.

Cancer cell

Normal cell

Figure 10.1

c) **Palliative surgery** may be needed even if the disease cannot be entirely removed in a curative operation. It may fix physical problems caused by the tumor, for example bleeding or obstruction of the intestine in the case of colon cancer. In this case the extent of surgery is limited to removing or bypassing the offending part. Additional removal is not attempted because attempting to do so might be risky or futile.

We will address more surgical issues in Chapter 11 on Surgery.

2) In **Radiation Therapy**, a sophisticated radiation delivery machine delivers radiation to the target area. The radiation for cancer treatment is produced by controlled radioactive chemicals. The tumor site is mapped carefully on a CAT scan picture. Then the area to be radiated (radiation field) is precisely drawn out and programmed into the radiation machine. The radiation machine delivers the treatment in small daily doses over several weeks until the total radiation dose required is reached. This total dose varies according to tumor site and purpose of treatment. Depending on the situation, the treatment takes several (5-7) weeks to complete. Sometimes it takes 10 days and rarely 1-3 days.

Radiation Therapy can be curative or palliative.

a) Curative radiation treatment intends to eradicate the cancer. This requires a higher dose and may cover the regional lymph nodes in addition to the tumor site. In some cases it is delivered simultaneously with chemotherapy for maximum benefit.

b) Palliative radiation treatment manages symptoms of advanced disease. Even if the cancer cannot be eradicated, tumors that are encroaching on nerves or blood vessels can be shrunk to reduce pain or bleeding. Pressure on airways can be alleviated to improve breathing. If tumors in the brain or in the vertebral column are causing local pressure, radiation can shrink the disease and relieve the pressure.

More information about Radiation Therapy is provided in Chapter 12.

3) Chemotherapy drugs kill immature cells by blocking the growth cycle of dividing cells. As antibiotics deal with infectious organisms like bacteria, chemotherapy drugs deal with cancer cells.

Chemotherapy can have different purposes:

a) Curative chemotherapy requires a specified number and combination of drugs. The number of treatments needed for a cure is established by clinical trials which are part of national guidelines. These standards change as new studies improve results with new drugs and schedules. Current standards for postoperative colon cancer chemotherapy are a total of 12 treatments spaced two weeks apart. Thirty years ago one year of chemotherapy was standard. As new standards have been developed, the number of postoperative Breast cancer chemotherapy treatments recommended has decreased from 12 to six to four over the last 40 years. As new drugs are developed they are incorporated into combinations that improve cure rates.

b) Radiosensitizing chemotherapy helps radiation therapy work better by making the target cells more sensitive to radiation therapy. Doses are smaller than regular chemotherapy doses because the purpose is to help radiation therapy, not be the main treatment. The treatment is coordinated with both the start and completion of radiation therapy.

c) Palliative chemotherapy alleviates symptoms by shrinking the tumor. If the tumor is causing pain or swelling, decreasing its volume can be a benefit even if the treatment is not curative.

d) **Chemotherapy can extend life in non-curative situations** by slowing tumor growth.

Chemotherapy is currently delivered mainly by an intravenous infusion. Depending on the drugs, this can take between a few minutes to several hours to several days via a portable continuous infusion pump. The infusion bag is connected directly into a vein in the arm or into a special device commonly called a port or portacath.

A few chemotherapy drugs are available in pill form. Many of the oral drugs are the newer agents that we will mention below. With oral chemotherapy you do not need to spend time in the Infusion Center. The pills, however, are not without side effects. More important, patients need to be fully compliant because chemotherapy pills often need to be taken daily with a week or so off between cycles. A missed dose or two can result in inadequate dosing of chemotherapy while misunderstanding the schedule can lead to dangerous overdosing. The advantage of intravenous chemotherapy is that the intended dose can be delivered accurately. But once it is in your body, it cannot be taken out. The advantage of the pills is that if complications arise, the treatment can be adjusted or suspended.

***

Thomas needed to take chemotherapy pills coordinated with his intravenous chemotherapy treatment that he received every three weeks. He was to take two pills daily for two weeks and the third week he would take no pills. The entire cycle was to be repeated six times. We drew out the schedule on calendars for him to take home and tried our best to make sure he understood. Two months later we got a refill request ahead of schedule. Thomas had run out of the pills because he had not stopped taking them during the prescribed break. We were all lucky that no harm was done. We have many safety checks when intravenous chemotherapy is administered in the infusion center, but we must rely on patients to follow the instructions at home for chemotherapy pills.

***

There are other ways to deliver chemotherapy in special situations. Chemotherapy ointments are used for some skin cancers. If cancer is in the lining of the space around the brain or spinal cord, chemotherapy can be injected into that space via a special device. Some treatments can be put into the urinary bladder. In some specific situations, chemotherapy can be put in the abdominal cavity.

Depending on the treatment plan, chemotherapy infusions are scheduled either every week or every two, three, or four weeks. They are usually delivered as a combination of drugs which complement each other's activity. There are standardized combinations for different kinds of cancer.

More information on Chemotherapy is provided in chapter 13.

These three above treatments manage cancers with a broad stroke: surgically removing the tumor, radiating it, or using chemotherapy to attack the cell division of cancer cells and some normal cells. The next few treatments attack specific targets on the cancer cells called hormone receptors, growth signals, or cancer-causing mutations.

4) Hormonal manipulation is used for hormone-sensitive tumors. Prostate cancer cells feed off testosterone, and some breast cancer cells feed off estrogen. Drugs have been developed to block the production of these hormones (anastrazole for breast cancer--brand name Arimidex), or to interfere with the hormone receptors (Nolvadex/Tamoxifen for breast cancer). This decreases cancer cell growth. While the cells don't immediately die, as with chemotherapy, they do shrivel up in the absence of their hormonal stimulation.

Hormone therapy can be used in
a) Curative situations. For example after lumpectomy+radiation, or mastectomy in breast cancer, five to ten years of hormone-blocking therapy improves cure rates.
b) Palliative therapy. When the disease has spread, interfering with hormone levels may still control it. If the hormone receptor is present on the breast cancer cell, it can be treated by hormone blocking agents even if the disease is growing in the bones or lungs. This will shrink the disease and can prolong life as long as the cell continues to respond to this blockade. Eventually the cancer cell will become resistant, and other treatments will be needed for disease control.

How will hormone therapy affect me?

Hormone therapy will not cause the chemotherapy-like side effects. The lack of the hormone will cause symptoms of hormone deprivation. Reducing testosterone and estrogen levels can decrease libido and cause hot flashes. Decreased hormone levels can contribute to thinning of the bones (osteoporosis), dry skin, and thinning hair. Some of the effects are reversible when the treatment finishes or is stopped.

5) In **Targeted therapy** drugs are designed against a specific target. The targets can be a growth receptor on the cell membrane or a cell messenger signal as described in the next section. The number of such targets is increasing every year. At present many of these drugs are being studied and used in relapsed disease, not in the early stages for cure. They have vastly increased the options for relapsed disease which often becomes resistant to chemotherapy with repeated treatments.

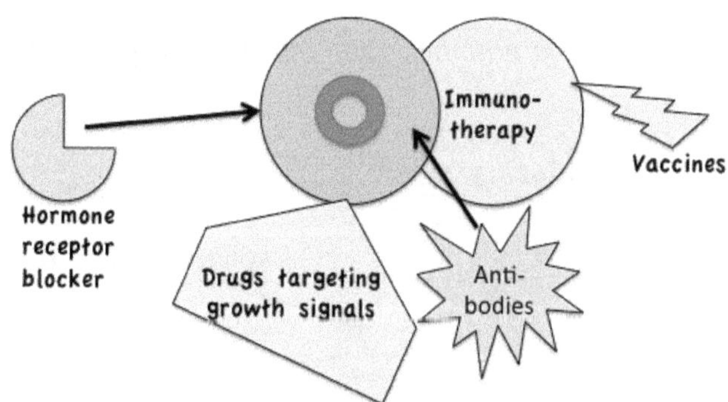

Targeted therapy:
Different targets, different pathways.

Figure 10.2

What is a receptor?

A receptor is a protein on the cell surface that acts as a messenger from the outside to the inside of the cell. Circulating messenger chemicals (like hormones or growth factors) bind to the external portion of the receptor on the cell membrane which is specific to that messenger. The binding causes changes inside the cell and sends a cascade of messenger chemicals to the nucleus of the cell. Cell division depends on an intricate system of signals that exist in the normal cell. When cell division is needed, some signals tell the cell to divide. This is similar to stepping on the accelerator to make the car move.

When the normal cells need to go into a dormant phase, other signals put the brakes on.

Cancer cells develop mutations or abnormalities in receptors that affect these signal pathways. When these signals are damaged, the brakes cannot be applied, the accelerator is unchecked, and the cells can divide uncontrollably. Oncologists have started to use drugs that target these damaged or mutated receptors, and such drugs will become more prevalent in the coming years.

Other signaling substances facilitate new blood vessel formation to supply the tumor. Tumors need new blood vessels to feed them. Some drugs that work to decrease these signals decrease the blood supply to the tumor which ultimately shrinks the supply of nutrients to the dividing cancer cells and starves them. An example of this treatment is Bevacizumab (brand name Avastin).

Another way the cancer cell survives is by turning off the programmed cell death that is present in normal cells. New drugs are available that counteract this turn-off and facilitate cancer cell death.

Where chemotherapy is like a hammer, targeted therapy works like a fine scalpel.

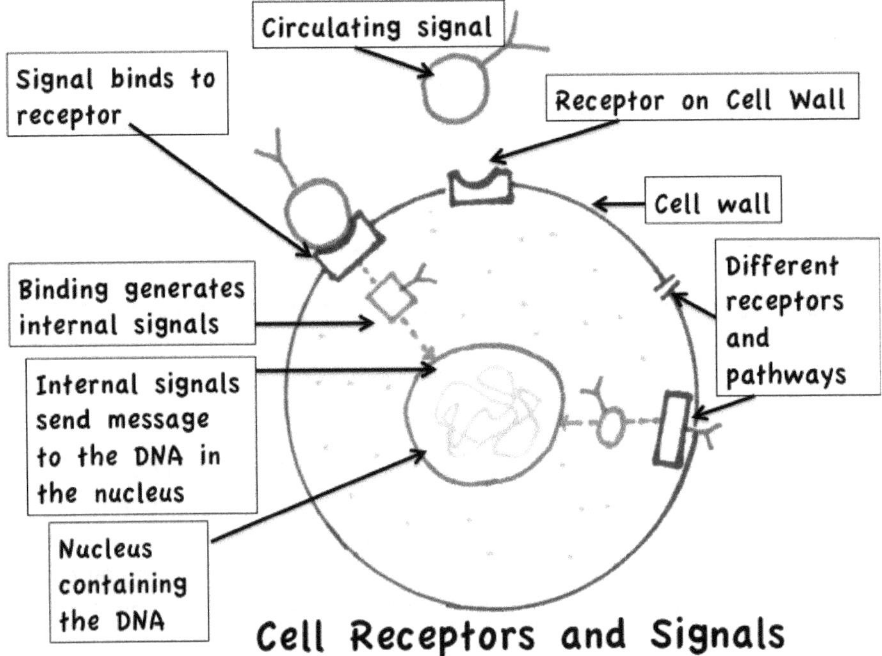

Figure 10.3

6) Immunotherapy is a way of harnessing the body's own immunity to attack the cancer cell. Cancer cells initially grow and thrive by escaping the body's scavenging system, as we discussed in Chapter 2. The cancer cell has ways of turning off the scavenging system which should normally attack it.

One kind of immunotherapy turns the body's own scavenging system back on. In another, antibodies are produced against the abnormal receptor that is helping cancer cell growth and are infused into the blood stream to find their target. The treatment needs to be given regularly to maintain the antibody levels at the effective saturation point. Trastuzumab (brand name Herceptin) acts against the her-2 neu receptor in breast and stomach cancer, and Rituximab (brand name Rituxan) binds to the CD20 protein on lymphoma cells.

Targeted and immune therapy minimizes the effect on normal tissue. Activating the immune system, however, can result in an attack on normal tissue, causing related side effects.

7) Vaccine therapy using the body's own immune system to produce immunity against the cancer cell has been tried. Unlike vaccines that act against infectious organisms, these vaccines are challenging to mass-produce. Each person's cancer cell can be different, and the immunity required against it needs to be individualized. At this time one vaccine is in commercial use. Prostate cancer cells harvested from the individual patient are sent to the company which produces a vaccine against that cell. The patient is then treated with a custom made vaccine.

8) Watchful waiting is possible for some cancers. If they are slow growing, they may not cause any symptoms for a while, and early treatment might not have any benefit over treatment given at a later date. For example chronic lymphocytic leukemia is often detected on a routine blood test. It does not need to be treated until the numbers grow rapidly or the disease causes other symptoms. Other cancers, like low-grade prostate cancers in older men, may not need to be treated at all.

Combination of choices:

All of these treatments may be used depending on different stages and situations. Sometimes the tumor needs to be removed first. Then follow-up treatment with radiation +/- chemotherapy +/- hormonal therapy is delivered. Sometimes radiation +/- chemotherapy is given before surgery to enable curative surgery. Some tumors are very sensitive to radiation/ chemotherapy and do not require surgery at all. This decision is individualized, depending on the patient, the kind of cancer, and the stage of disease.

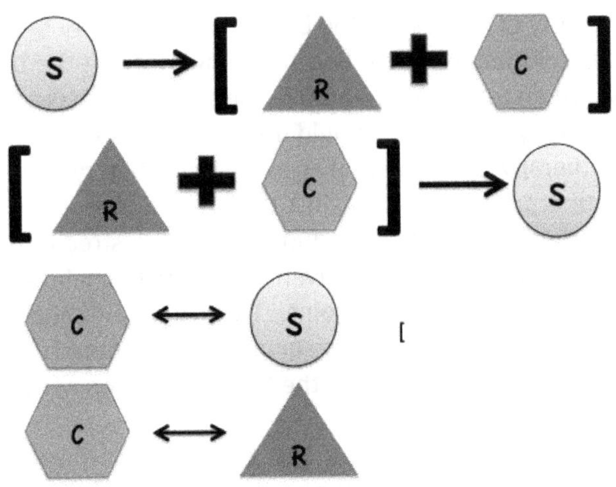

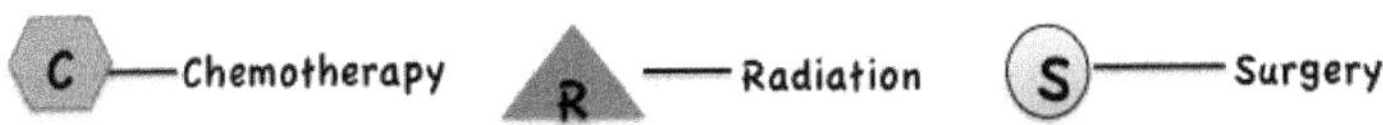

Figure 10.4 Treatment Sequence

Am I strong enough to take all this treatment?

Treatment is tailored to each person's Performance Status.

Why is Performance status important?

Even if the treatment is curative, when a person is so debilitated by age or other illnesses, they may find the side effects of treatment overwhelming. Can they undergo the whole course of treatment? Will they be terminally harmed by the treatment? Is the cure worse than the disease? If the patient is debilitated, treatment is not going to be effective in improving their quality of life. Complications of treatment may possibly shorten it.

On the other hand, if the cause of the weakness is the cancer itself, the treatment, however harsh, may ultimately improve their condition by shrinking the disease. It may seem counter intuitive to start strong chemotherapy when the person is very weak. They might not, however, get better without starting the treatment.

What is Performance Status? (PS)

Two objective scales, the Karnofsky scale and the ECOG scale, measure physical conditioning and the ability to carry out Activities of Daily Living (ADLs). The better your Performance Status, the better able you are to withstand treatment.

Can I improve my Performance Status?

You can improve some factors of your performance status, and some you cannot. You can try to improve your nutrition and hydration. Physical therapy can improve exercise conditioning. Control of pain and mental health support can help functioning. You may not be able to improve other chronic conditions like heart disease.

The act of choosing treatment is a tradeoff between the benefit and the side effects. Treatment choices are carefully considered before starting treatment. While the wait for treatment to begin can be excruciating, it takes time to gather all the necessary information to go down the right path.

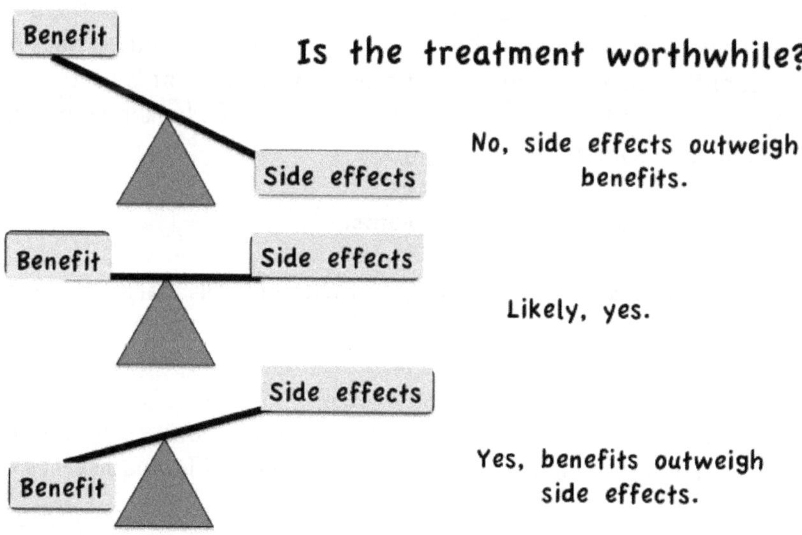

Figure 10.5

What is a Bone Marrow Transplant?

Normal blood cells are produced in the bone marrow. Normal blood cells have a life span from a few days to up to three months. Stem cells are precursor cells and act as a reservoir from which new, mature cells develop. These new, mature cells then go into circulation to replace the old ones. As chemotherapy circulates through the bone marrow, normal blood cell production is interrupted, but adequate numbers of stem cells are present to replace the normal cells in a few days.

When a very high dose of chemotherapy is needed to wipe out the cancer cells all at once, as in cancers affecting the blood or bone marrow like leukemia, the normal stem cells are wiped out as well. Not enough stem cells are left over to replace the lost cells. In preparation for the high dose chemotherapy, normal stem cells are harvested from the blood stream before the high dose chemotherapy, stored, and infused back into the patient to regrow normal blood cells. This treatment is used mainly for those cancers that originate in the bone marrow: leukemia, multiple myeloma, and, sometimes, lymphomas.

There are two main types of transplants.

Autologous transplants use the patient's own stem cells that are harvested and stored before the high dose chemotherapy.

Allogeneic transplants use donor stem cells.

Which one is better? The kind of stem cells, self or donor, is determined by the kind of disease being treated. Each is used in different diseases and situations.

In the past actual bone marrow was harvested, stored, and re-infused. Modern stem cell collection techniques allow the stem cells to be gathered from the blood stream by circulating the blood through a special machine. This has made it easier on the patient.

What is personalized medicine?

All treatment decisions are personalized for the type of cancer, the stage, and the condition of the patient. When the decision to proceed with chemotherapy is made, the organ of origin and the stage determines the choice of drugs. The doses are tailored to the patient's Body Surface Area (BSA) which is calculated from their height and body weight. A five foot 90 pound woman will not get the same total dose as the six foot 200 pound man, but the ratio of the chemotherapy to their body's volume is standardized and will be the same. At this time the same combination of drugs is given for all post-operative patients with colon cancer, regardless of the characteristics of the cell or mutations on their cell walls. Chemotherapy is one big hammer which will miss the nail in some patients or hammer it through the wood in others.

Precision medicine is a process of matching the target and the drug rather than the disease and the drug.

As we learn more about the genetic changes in the cancer cell and mutations in its receptors, drugs will be designed to attack those changes without attacking all the surrounding cells. We will be able to selectively choose the treatment appropriate to the target. In time the organ of origin may become less important.

Gene mutation and receptor analyses test for targets for which drugs have already been developed and are commercially available in the United States. They have been incorporated into standardized treatment plans. This avenue of treatment can be accessed from any cancer treatment facility and is not limited to research facilities.

Large-scale gene mapping can be done in University-based cancer centers, but it is useful mainly for research purposes at this time. Without drugs to attack the uncovered targets, this work belongs in the research arena. The expense and value added by using gene mapping in the mainstream oncology population is unclear at this time.

Neal and Mona had heard the evening news report on the National Lung Cancer Society which was having its annual meeting that week. There was a press release about a promising new drug for lung cancer. The preliminary results of the Phase 1 trial had been presented at the conference, but it would be several more years before the results were proven in larger studies and the treatment became available. Neal's oncologist explained that the drug reported on the evening news would not be ready in time to treat Neal.

Promising preliminary studies often make the evening news during large cancer conferences. If some drugs appear really promising, one way to be treated with them is to enroll in a clinical trial if one is available.

In the US, the National Cancer Institute maintains a list of available clinical trials on its website. Your oncologist can help you decide if a clinical trial is appropriate.

Action Plan: Questions to ask...

- Can I improve my Performance Status?
- What is my Stage?
- Is this the best treatment for me? Should I enroll in a clinical trial?
- Will I see a Nutritionist during treatment? What should I eat? What should I avoid?
- Do I need Physical Therapy? Oxygen? Pain Management?
- Can I get a Flu shot?
- Can I have dental work?
- Do I need to stay away from crowds?
- Can I work during treatments? Should I bring someone with me for the treatments?

Glossary of terms:

- Curative=Treatment that will eradicate cancer cells completely.
- Non-curative, or Life- extending=Treatment that will not cure the disease but will slow disease growth.
- Palliative=Treatment that intends to alleviate symptoms related to the tumor.
- Adjuvant Treatment=Treatment added *after* main curative treatment to improve cure rates.
- Neoadjuvant Treatment=Treatment given *before* main curative treatment to improve cure rates.

11. Surgery 101

Neal and Mona consult with the chest surgeon thinking that removal of the tumor would be the first step. Thirty years ago they would have been correct.

Surgery used to be the mainstay of treatment, and for many cancers it still is. We have come a long way since the days when, because there were few other available curative treatments, aggressive radical surgery was considered the only possible cure for cancer. The most notable example of radical surgery is the radical mastectomy.

The first radical mastectomy in the United States was performed in 1882 by Dr. William Halstead who was the Chief of Surgery at the Johns Hopkins University School of Medicine in Baltimore, Maryland, and championed this approach. Halstead's operation for breast cancer pursued cure by removing the breast, the surrounding lymph nodes, the muscles of the chest wall, and anything else that might be suspect. The extent of the surgery led to many postoperative complications. Severe scarring limited movement of the arm. Extensive lymph node removal resulted in swelling (lymphedema) as the lymph fluid backed up into the arm. Nevertheless, the radical mastectomy remained the main treatment for breast cancer in the US until the 1970s. In spite of the aggressive removal of surrounding tissue, this radical surgery was not more curative than a less invasive simple mastectomy. Eventually surgery for breast cancer was limited to the lump itself and a single lymph node. We are on our way, in selected situations, to avoiding lymph node removal altogether.

Combining surgery with radiation and chemotherapy either before or after surgery has enabled a smaller, less-debilitating operation for many other cancers.

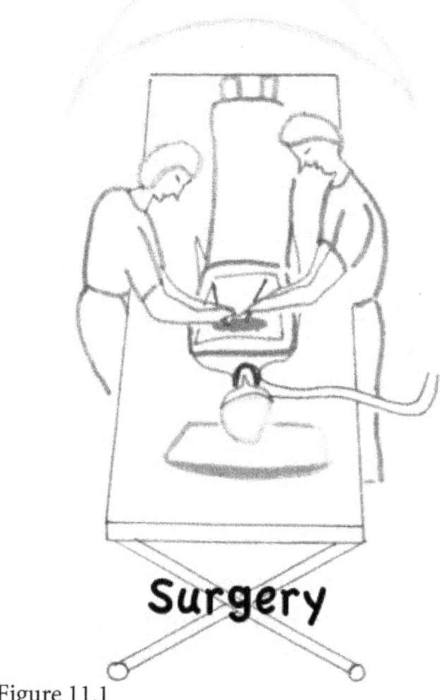

Figure 11.1

What is the role of Surgery?

* Surgery may be needed for **diagnosis.** If a biopsy is not easily obtained by an external procedure, a limited surgery can be performed to obtain tissue. Even in advanced disease, when the tumors cannot be completely removed, tissue is still required to confirm the nature of the cancer cell.

* **For cure**: In many cancers, for example kidney cancer, surgery remains the only curative mode of treatment. In order for surgery to be curative, the cancer needs to be limited to the involved organ or a limited surgical area. It cannot be present elsewhere in the body. Scans done before an operation ensure there is no visible cancer in other parts of the body (distant disease). The entire tumor must be removed (resection), otherwise the remaining cancer cells will grow back, make more tumors, and the surgery will eventually be unsuccessful. After the operation, the pathologist makes sure that an adequate margin of clean tissue exists around the resected tumor. In some situations additional surgery to remove extra tissue is required to clean up the margins. Sometimes this confirmation can be given during an operation when the pathologist takes a "frozen section" while you are on the operating table and before the slides are processed.

* **Palliative Surgery:** If extensive disease is found during the operation and the goal of cure cannot be achieved, the surgery is either stopped or changed to a palliative operation. Even if the cancer cannot be removed in its entirety, surgery may be required to fix local problems. The physical presence of the tumor can cause blockage of the intestine or bleeding that cannot be fixed without removal of the offending tumor. A tumor in the spinal column may be pressing upon the spinal cord. Surgery on the offending vertebra may be needed for decompression.

Palliative surgery can be performed as necessary, as and when symptoms arise. The number of times surgery is undertaken will depend on the overall condition of the patient, life expectancy at that point, and whether surgery can improve the quality of life. The goal of treatment always needs to be considered before proceeding. Is the surgery going to make life longer or better?

* **Debulking surgery**, or removal of as much of the tumor as possible, is an accepted procedure in a few varieties of cancer. Even if surgery does not make the person cancer free, taking out most of the tumor increases the success rate for the chemotherapy or immunotherapy that will occur afterwards. This is true, however, of only a few cancers like ovarian cancer and kidney cancer.

What is removed in curative surgery?

Commonly curative surgery removes the **primary tumor,** the **margin** of non-cancerous tissue surrounding the tumor, and **lymph nodes** that produce infection-fighting cells for that area. Sometimes (occasionally) only part of the organ needs to be removed and the rest of it will continue to function. If removing only the involved portion of the organ can preserve it, every effort is made to do so. For example a small kidney tumor may only require partial removal of the kidney, or a small lung tumor may only require removal of the affected portion of the lung.

Some questions can arise when we discuss whether surgery is an option for treatment.

What are lymph nodes? Why are the lymph nodes removed?

As we discussed earlier in Chapter 7 (Staging), lymph nodes are collections of immunity-processing cells that act as filters for particles that your body does not recognize as its own. Some of these particles are cancer cells. Each area of the body is served by its own group of lymph nodes. Tissue fluid around the cells travels through a system of lymph ducts or lymphatic vessels to the local lymph nodes. If the lymph nodes detect an infection or inflammation, they go into action to fight it. You can feel the lymph nodes in the neck swell up when you have an infection in the throat. When there is a tumor, cancer cells can travel to that area's lymph nodes. Checking those lymph nodes for cancer cells is necessary to correctly stage, or map out, where the cancer is located, because the treatment can change depending on the stage of the cancer.

Why does lymph node surgery cause lymphedema?

If a large number of lymph nodes need to be surgically removed, lymph drainage from that area can be slowed. This can lead to swelling or lymphedema and is similar to a traffic back up on the highway when construction narrows the lanes available for use. Removal of lymph nodes from the armpit in breast cancer surgery can lead to swelling in that arm.

What is a sentinel lymph node biopsy?

In trying to reduce the ill effects of radical surgery, we are also trying to reduce the after effects of radical lymph node dissection (or removal). Because there are many scattered lymph nodes downstream from a tumor, surgeons need to remove all of the local lymph nodes that could harbor cancer cells that escaped from the tumor. If only we had a map of the path cancer cells might take from the tumor to the lymph node that serves it we wouldn't have to remove so many lymph nodes.

Sentinel lymph node mapping attempts to answer this question. A dye is injected at the site of the tumor. The sentinel lymph node is the one that the dye first travels to, and that is the one that is removed. If any other lymph nodes in the area take up the dye, they are removed as well. As a result of this procedure, we have been able to move away from a more extensive, or

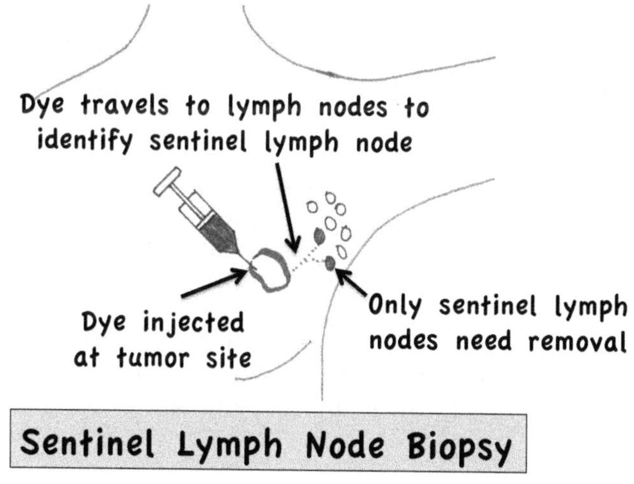

Figure 11.2

radical, lymph node dissection. (See Figure 11.2). Sentinel lymph node biopsy is now routinely done in breast cancer and melanoma surgery.

Sentinel lymph node mapping is still being evaluated for other cancers. Some areas are not amenable to this procedure for technical reasons. In some areas of the body the lymph can drain in many different directions. The single sentinel lymph node may not be the only recipient of cancer cells, and a more complete dissection may be required as in head and neck cancers.

If they take out all my lymph nodes, do I have any left?

Lymph nodes are not a single organ but collections of lymph tissue throughout the body. The largest such collection is in the spleen, but there are innumerable lymph nodes throughout the body. Plenty of lymph nodes are left for processing immunity after some are removed.

The surgeon said the surgery was successful, and they got all the cancer out. Why do I need more treatment with radiation and chemotherapy?

Taking out the tumor is the first step towards the cure. Preventing it from returning is the second step. We need both steps for success. In American Professional Football rules, both feet need to be inside the lines to be called a completed pass. The risk of a relapse (or recurrence) increases with the size of the primary tumor, any involvement of the lymph nodes, infiltration of the tumor into the surrounding tissue, and the nature of the cancer cell. Postoperative treatment intends to kill off any hiding cancer cells and prevent them from showing up in the years ahead as new tumors. Not all cancers need or benefit from postoperative treatment. Treatment is only offered if benefit has been proven through clinical studies. If there is no proven benefit, treatment is not offered, even if the risk of relapse is significant. All treatment causes side effects, and we do not want to inflict side effects without proven benefit.

Why do I need all this treatment, surgery, radiation AND chemotherapy? Is my situation serious?

Postoperative treatment is offered to maximize cures by preventing relapses. After curative surgery, the recommendation for postoperative treatment is based upon risk of relapse and the proven benefit in decreasing that risk. This does not imply that your situation is serious or dire. It does mean that cure rates can be improved with additional treatment.

Why can't we wait to see if the cancer relapses, and then use radiation and chemotherapy afterwards?

For most cancers the best chance of a cure is during the first set of treatments. After a relapse, repeat curative operations in most cancers are usually not feasible for technical reasons. A relapse may show up in a distant site as a metastasis. In addition, the cancer cell can evolve into a more resistant cell in relapses, and curative treatment may not then be possible. We front-load the treatment options for cure at first pass. Not everyone would relapse if they did not undergo postoperative treatment, but we do not have the tests to identify only those patients who need and will benefit from additional treatment at present. Some predictive tests have been developed for some cancers, like the Oncotype DX score in breast cancer. This helps us separate patients who have a high risk of relapse from those with a low risk. Only those patients at high risk of relapse receive chemotherapy. As more such tests are developed, we will be better able to select patients for postoperative treatment.

Why can't we just cut out the spots in my liver when we remove my lung tumor?

Most cancer cells get to the distant site through circulation in the blood or lymph stream. Because cancer cells remain in circulation, they are moving targets. New cancerous spots will appear as the circulating cells find a home and grow into tumors. This makes it impossible to go after every distant spot. This explains why heroic surgery is not offered when disease has spread. It would be futile.

There are some exceptions to this rule in a limited number of situations, but strict guidelines exist to avoid surgery that would not benefit the patient.

My neighbor had Stage 4 colon cancer, and they took out the spots on her liver along with half her colon.

That is one of the exceptions to the above rule. In a very limited number of situations, if a very small number of spots exist in only one portion of the liver, removal of that portion of the liver improves survival in colon cancer. Often removal of the colon is followed by postoperative chemotherapy. If no new disease shows itself elsewhere after the initial chemotherapy, doctors will undertake resection of the spots on the liver. If new disease shows up in that interval, then liver resection is not attempted. The disease has declared itself to be a "spreader;" more surgery is not going to be useful.

Why can't I have a liver transplant if the cancer has spread to my liver?

Circulating cancer cells pose a huge problem. They will find a home in the transplanted organ or elsewhere, and the organ transplant itself will not be life saving. The goal of cure will not be achieved.

The exception is cancer of the liver itself (not cancer that has spread to the liver). Ideally the involved portion of the liver can be removed leaving adequate healthy liver. When that is not technically feasible, a liver transplant is an option.

Does doing surgery cause the cancer to spread?

Patients do have this question because they know someone who had surgery and developed distant disease six months later. Oncologists and surgeons used to believe that because cancer cells have the opportunity to spread by the lymph or blood vessels at any time prior to the surgery, surgery itself did not cause the cancer to spread.

As we gain more understanding of the immune reaction to surgery, however, we are beginning to realize that the trauma of surgery may cause changes in immunity as well as changes in the lining of blood vessels. This change may facilitate the spread of cancer cells. That doesn't mean patients should not undertake curative surgery. You can discuss with your surgeon whether it would be safe and reasonable to use an anti-inflammatory drug pre-operatively. More research is required into modifying the body's immune response to surgery.

What are the newer techniques for surgery?

Not all cancer operations require an open operation. Some tumors can be removed laparoscopically in a process whereby small tubes and cameras are introduced into the body through several small incisions. Some operations are being done with the assistance of special robots that can allow more manipulation of the organ with smaller incisions.

The important point is that the operation is clean, that the cancer cells cannot be spilled into the body cavity. In a technique of uterine fibroid removal called morcellation, the fibroid is pulverized into small pieces through a laparoscopic procedure and the pieces sucked out. This procedure is done for benign fibroids. The risk is that if cancer cells are found in the pieces afterwards, it was not a clean cancer operation. When a newer technique is suggested to you, make sure that it does not carry the risk of letting cancer cells escape.

Should *Neal* have an operation? In order to have a curative operation, the tumor has to be cleanly and entirely removed without leaving any cancer cells behind. Since Neal's tumor involves the local lymph nodes and is located in an area where it would be difficult to remove cleanly, surgery would not be recommended as the first approach. Neal will meet with the Radiation Oncologist and Medical Oncologist to discuss radiation and chemotherapy.

Action Plan:

- Ask if surgery is the standard first approach for your stage of cancer.
- If yes, will any intervention improve the post surgical outcome?
- If yes, will it likely be followed by additional treatment?
- If not, is surgery planned after other treatment to shrink the disease?
- If you have metastatic disease, would you be a candidate for surgery at a later point?

12. Radiation Therapy 101

Neal is not a candidate for surgery at this time. His tumor is too large and too close to vital blood vessels to enable a safe and clean removal. Curative treatment is still possible with a combination of radiation and chemotherapy. Neal and Mona consult with the Radiation Oncologist as part of his treatment planning. What should they expect?

Firstly, what is radiation?

Radiation is a form of energy travelling through space, originating from a specific source. Different kinds of energy travel at their own unique wavelengths. The sun gives us light energy and ultraviolet radiation. Radiation is present in our natural environment in radioactive elements like radium and uranium. It can be produced artificially for medical reasons like X rays that are used in scanners for diagnosis. Ionizing radiation causes damage to tissue, and exposure needs to be limited to safe doses. When this energy is directed in a controlled fashion onto the tumor, it is used in the treatment of cancer.

A **Radiation Oncologist** is a cancer specialist who treats cancer with radiation therapy. Some cancers are treated exclusively with radiation therapy and others are combined with chemotherapy. Combination treatment with chemotherapy can occur either simultaneously or sequentially or both. The treatment is delivered in small daily doses until the total dose is reached. The Radiation Oncologist prescribes the dose of radiation required to treat the disease (per established standards). Doses for cure are higher than doses that are palliative. Since the daily dose is limited for safety reasons, curative treatment takes longer to complete.

Cancers that are commonly treated with radiation therapy are cancers of the breast, the oral cavity and throat, the esophagus or food pipe, the lung, the rectum and the prostate, and lymphomas (cancers of the lymph glands themselves, not cancer that has spread to the lymph glands).

How does radiation kill cancer cells?

Radiation damages the DNA (genetic material) of the cell either directly or indirectly by creating ionized particles within the cell. A cancer cell needs to divide its DNA in order to keep growing, and the damaged DNA cannot divide. Unfortunately, some normal cells in the path of the radiation are also damaged. The area becomes inflamed and swollen while the body copes with the damaged normal cells. The required daily treatment does not allow for the inflammation to subside until the entire course of treatment is over. Recovery then takes a few weeks.

Treatment Planning:

The first session with the Radiation Oncologist is the longest one. The tumor site is mapped carefully on a CAT scan picture, and the area to be radiated (radiation field) is carefully drawn out and programmed into the radiation machine. The Radiation Oncologist and the physicist calculate the delivery angles and the depth of penetration of the radiation beam required to reach the target tissues. They position the patient on the treatment table and mark (tattoo) the area to be radiated with very small ink dots. These dots are permanent but barely visible. The radiation machine delivers treatment in programmed daily doses. It takes several weeks until the total radiation dose required is reached. This total dose varies according to tumor site and reason for treatment.

After the initial treatment planning session, subsequent daily treatments are short visits that include a quick check-up and positioning on the radiation table. The radiation therapist sees you every day for the treatment, the nurse is available for any questions, and the doctor sees you once a week for a check-up and to answer any questions.

How is the treatment delivered?

Radiation can be delivered in a variety of ways depending on the cancer being treated. Lung cancer treatment will require different techniques than Skin cancer or cancer of the cervix.

* **External beam radiation (EBRT)** is the most common, and it is delivered as described above.

* **Brachytherapy** is a technique developed to deliver radiation internally to

the target organ via radioactive needles. The seeds, or needles, are placed inside the tumor site by an applicator when you are under anesthesia. The applicator is removed, but the seeds or needles stay in place. For some treatments the needles are removed at a later date. At other times they can stay in place. This technique is used mainly to deliver radiation directly to the prostate gland or the cervix. Other cancers are occasionally treated with this method.

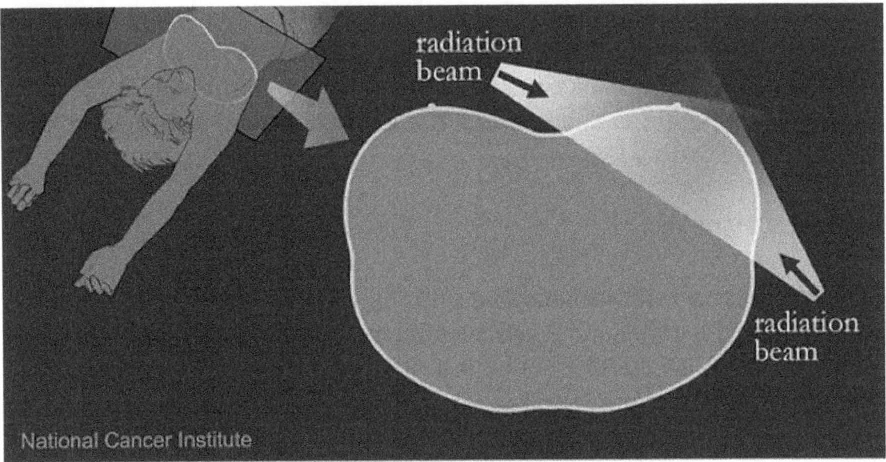

Illustrator: Don Bliss

Figure 12.1

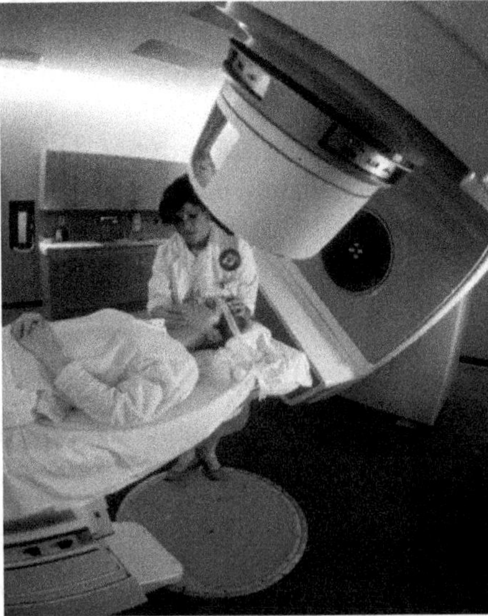

Patient being positioned on Radiation Machine

Courtesy: NCI
Photographer: Mark Anderson

Figure 12.2

* **Superficial skin radiation** machines deliver treatment to skin cancers. This form of radiation does not need to penetrate far into the body.

* **IMRT or Intensity Modulated Radiation Therapy** is delivered by special machines that are currently available only at a few radiation centers. IMRT allows the Radiation Oncologist to pinpoint the tumor and draw the radiation area more tightly around the target organ so that it does not affect too much of the surrounding tissue. It is much more expensive than standard EBRT, and the relative improvement in outcomes is still being established.

* **Intraoperative radiotherapy** is sometimes given directly to a tumor during an operation. The normal organs are moved out of the way and shielded with a special apron. After the radiation is delivered, the organs are put back in place. This way the tumor site can get a large dose of radiation without affecting the surrounding organs.

* **Stereotactic Radiosurgery/ Gamma knife/ Cyber knife** are techniques to deliver a high dose of treatment to a small area in a single setting. No cutting or surgery is involved. This method is often used when tumors relapse and repeat treatments are needed--most commonly in the brain.

* **Radiopharmaceuticals** are radioactive compounds injected into the blood stream which travel to the desired locations and can deliver radiation to multiple sites at one time. When cancer has spread to different bones, the radioactive chemical is given by intravenous infusion, circulates, and is taken up by the affected spots. This method delivers radiation therapy to all of the spots at the same time in one treatment. Radioactive iodine which is selectively taken up by thyroid tissue and treats thyroid cancer is another example.

How do they know the treatment is working?

During the course of radiation therapy, doctors periodically perform CT scans on the tumor to make sure it is not growing while they are treating it. There is no formal assessment that includes measurements. The full response to the treatments may not be noted for some time because the radiation can work slowly. It can continue to shrink the tumor for weeks after the treatment is finished. Because the radiation acts as an irritant, the area targeted gets inflamed and swollen, and accurate measurement of the tumor is difficult to obtain until the inflammation has decreased. That is why follow-up scans are not scheduled for six to eight weeks after the treatment is completed.

Will radiation treatment make me feel sick? When will I start feeling sick?

Controlled radiation delivery as it is done for treatment is different from an accidental exposure due to a nuclear accident when the whole body is exposed to a massive dose all at one time. The small daily doses for treatment will not make you instantly sick.

The side effects will depend on the area being targeted, and they will start building up two to three weeks after treatment begins. They will continue to intensify until the end of the treatment. Although treatment can eventually become uncomfortable, it is usually not interrupted, because each day's treatment builds on the effect of the previous one.

What side effects can I expect?

The side effects will depend on which organ is being radiated.

- **Prostate and rectum** radiation therapy causes diarrhea and burning with urination and possible sores around the bottom.
- **Oral Cavity, throat, and esophagus** (food pipe) radiation causes sores in the mouth and throat with pain and difficulty swallowing. This can result in malnutrition and dehydration.
- **Lung radiation** can cause inflammation of the food pipe when the food pipe is within the target radiation field. It can also cause delayed inflammation and scarring of the lung.
- **Breast radiation** can cause some skin redness and soreness.

Will the treatment make me feel tired?

Yes, but it will not do this immediately. You will experience fatigue as the treatment proceeds through its course. If the target area involves major bones, like the pelvis, spine or breastbone, it can affect blood cell production in the marrow of those bones. As the blood cell production is decreased, fewer circulating red cells transport oxygen. This will cause your body to tire easily. Radiation can also cause fatigue without low blood counts because it causes inflammation. The damaged cells release chemicals that contribute to fatigue.

Will radiation therapy cause hair loss?

Radiation therapy to the brain can cause hair loss because hair follicles in the scalp are damaged. Radiation to the face or neck can decrease facial hair. Radiation to other parts of the body does not cause general hair loss.

If my cancer returns, can I get radiation treatment again?

Yes, but only if your cancer returns in a different spot. Radiation therapy has several limitations. There is a limit on how much radiation a specific part of your body can receive and there is a lifetime memory of the radiation received in the radiated tissue. Doses that are initially delivered for cure are close to that lifetime total, and there is very little margin for retreatment if the tumor recurs in the same spot. A repeat course of radiation to the same spot will likely exceed the safe dose. This can be very risky, and doctors will only undertake it if there is no other option. Exceeding the total recommended dose to an area carries the risk of tissue breakdown, and, depending on the location, this can severely damage the organ involved.

If the cancer relapses in a different part of your body, however, it can be treated with radiation without difficulty.

How can I minimize side effects?

You will be given instructions specific to the area being radiated.

* **Mouth Care** is necessary when treating the oral cavity and throat. Radiation can affect the production of saliva and predispose the teeth to decay. Doctors recommend a dental check-up before treatment starts to take care of any urgent issues. Special rinses and fluoride treatments will help you take care of your teeth and gums. You may develop thrush (a fungal infection) and will need special mouthwashes and anti-fungal medication

* **Skin care** will be necessary as the treatment continues. If you develop redness or soreness, ointments like aquaphor are available. If your skin becomes raw and breaks down, ointments like Silvadene will be recommended. Do not use the ointments before your daily treatment because they can interfere with the penetration of radiation.

* **Nutrition and Hydration:** Minimize dehydration and malnourishment by actively increasing the amount of liquids that you take in. If eating solid food becomes difficult, eat more soft foods like pasta or pureed foods, and supplement them with nutrition drinks or frappes. Ask to see a nutritionist, and monitor your weight closely.

My throat is really sore, and it is painful to swallow. What can I do?

If your throat or food pipe is being radiated, it becomes inflamed and sore, and you may find it difficult to consume the amount of food or water you need. If you are becoming dehydrated and unable to keep up with your required intake by mouth, you may need to get liquids and other nourishment through intravenous hydration. Sometimes a temporary feeding tube, which can deliver liquid nourishment into the stomach, may be needed. There are several ways of delivering stomach-feeding tubes, and the choice will depend on your treatment center. One, the nasogastric (nasal) tube, is fed into the stomach by introducing it through the nose. The second, a gastric (stomach) tube, is placed through the abdominal wall directly into the stomach. Each has pros and cons. The nasal tube is placed by a nurse and does not require a surgical procedure, but it is very thin because it has to pass through your nose into your stomach. It stays there until it is not needed anymore. It gets clogged easily and often needs to be replaced. You cannot crush medication tablets and deliver them through a nasal tube. The gastric tube is placed through the abdominal wall in a procedure carried out in the Interventional Radiology suite or the Minor Surgery suite. You will need local anesthesia and some instruction on care of the tube. The tube can be capped and used as needed for liquid nutrition, hydration, and crushed tablets. It does not prevent swallowing of regular food by mouth, and it can be removed when treatment is complete and it is no longer needed.

Do I need to stay away from children or pregnant women?

Your radiation stays within your own body. You are not contagious, and you do not "glow in the dark." In some treatments (e.g. brachytherapy) special precautions do need to be taken, but standard treatments do not require isolation.

Can I travel when I am getting treatment?

Treatment is planned to take several weeks at a time, and it is important not to interrupt it if at all possible. Each day's treatment builds on the previous day's, and unnecessary interruption can affect the benefit of the radiation. If treatment has to be interrupted for medical reasons, the number of treatments can be made up at the end.

Treatments are scheduled from Monday to Friday, usually at the same time each day. Weekend treatments are only scheduled for emergencies. If treatment is being combined with chemotherapy, that schedule is coordinated with the Infusion Center and Medical Oncologist.

Neal's treatment plan...

Since Neal will require radiation treatments for his lung cancer, a treatment planning session is scheduled for him. He will also see a nutritionist who will advise him on how he can keep up with his nourishment and hydration. The cancer center will also make sure he can schedule rides to get to the center when he doesn't feel well enough to drive himself. If Neal cannot find rides for all his treatments, volunteers in the community may be able to help him out.

Action Plan:

- Ask if radiation therapy is part of a standard treatment plan.
- Will chemotherapy be given simultaneously? Or later?
- Is surgery planned for the future?
- Is there help with daily transportation if you need it?
- Ask to see a nutritionist.
- Should you see a dentist?
- Clear your schedule for the duration of treatment.

13. Chemotherapy 101

Neal is seen by a Medical Oncologist who is a cancer doctor specializing in chemotherapy. A Radiation Oncologist also reviews his case, and together they decide that he will need chemotherapy and radiation therapy simultaneously.

In this chapter we will review information, questions, and concerns about chemotherapy.

What is Chemotherapy?

Chemotherapy refers to a group of drugs or medications that damage both normal and cancerous cells by interrupting their cell division process. Cancer cells are constantly dividing and are more vulnerable to chemotherapy than normal cells. Normal cells divide intermittently to replace older cells, but they go through a dormant phase between cell division when they are not vulnerable to chemotherapy. Only a fraction of the body's normal cells is dividing at any time, and only a fraction of them is vulnerable to chemotherapy.

What is a Cycle of Chemotherapy?

A cycle of chemotherapy is a schedule of chemotherapy given at a predetermined interval. The interval varies from two to four weeks, and it creates a pattern of a nadir, or low point, of blood counts followed by recovery. The chemotherapy itself can be administered every week or every two, three, or four weeks (See Figure 13.1). Blood tests determine what happens throughout the whole cycle so that doctors can make adjustments, if needed, to the next cycle. Treatment doses and intervals can sometimes be changed to address any issues. Injections to boost blood production may be added for the next cycle. Additional nausea medicines or intravenous fluids may also be needed.

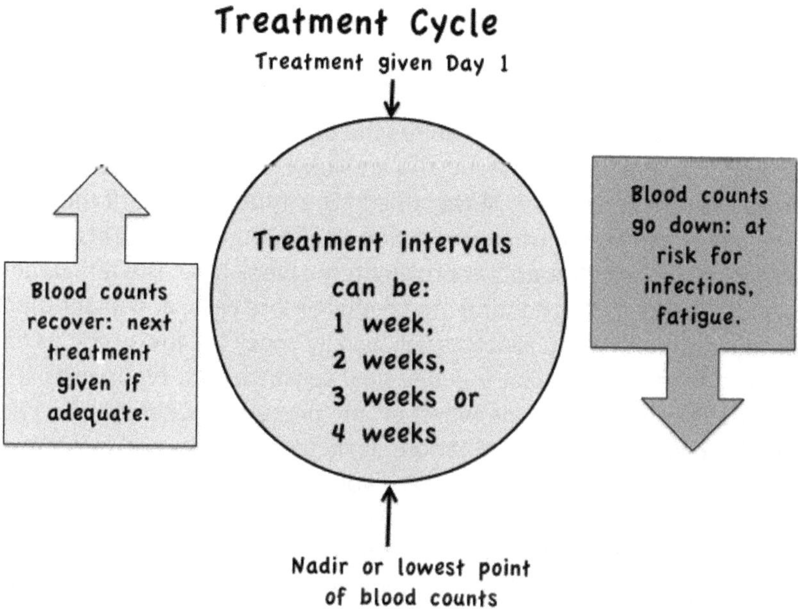

Figure 13.1

What happens with each chemotherapy visit?

Before each treatment you will have a set of blood tests. They may be done on the day before or on the same day as your chemotherapy depending on the practice at your center, your schedule, and your doctor's orders. This is to ensure your blood-count numbers are in the safe zone when you receive chemotherapy. You will have a check up to make sure you are physically able to undergo the current treatment and have had no earlier complications. Adjustments to the doses, or the plan, can be made at this time. At a scheduled time, you will come to the infusion suite where the infusion nurse and pharmacist will review your information and the doctor's orders again. The chemotherapy drugs are mixed in the infusion bag after this check. Anti-nausea medications may be given by mouth or through your vein followed by the chemotherapy drugs. The infusion can take from a few minutes to a few hours. Because the anti-nausea medications can make you drowsy, it is better to have someone take you home, especially the first time. Chemotherapy suites have accommodations for privacy as well as interaction. Often, since people come regularly on the same schedule, they develop friendships with the nurses and their fellow patients and enjoy some interaction. At other times patients who are having difficulty or want to work or take a nap can draw the curtains or be accommodated in a private room.

What are the side effects of chemotherapy?

Low blood counts: Normal blood cells consist of white cells, red cells, and platelets, and they are being continuously produced in the bone marrow from the precursor or stem cells. This requires the duplication and division of their genetic material. Precursor or stem cells are vulnerable to chemotherapy in a similar way as cancer cells are. At the time of the infusion some of the normal cells are killed, and the normal production line is interrupted. This causes a drop in normal blood cell counts approximately a week later. The remainder of the normal precursor cells continue to produce more cells, and in another 10 days production catches up. Doctors will usually check the low point, or nadir count, after the first treatment to judge how sensitive your blood cells are to the treatment. They will decide whether any precautions need to be taken. A **low white cell count** makes you more likely to get fevers and infections. A **low red cell count**, or anemia, can make you feel tired or short of breath. A **low platelet count** can make you bruise or bleed more easily. Depending on the combination of drugs in your chemotherapy mix, some of these effects can be more or less noticeable. If you get any of these side effects, tell your doctor or nurse so they can be treated and you can continue with the planned chemotherapy. You may need antibiotics if you develop a fever or a blood transfusion if your red cell count is too low. Dose adjustments or schedule adjustments are made accordingly. If you need to stay on schedule, you may be started on an injection the day after chemotherapy to speed up the recovery of the white cells.

Fatigue is not entirely due to low blood counts. It may be due to the release of cytokines which are messenger chemicals that may be released as the chemotherapy works.

Shallow ulcers of the mouth can occur because of the loss of the inner lining cells of the mouth. The mouth bacteria can change and a fungal infection can develop. This will need treatment with special mouthwashes or antifungal medication.

Nausea is generally controlled well with medications. Anti-nausea medications are taken before, during, and after chemotherapy. Please follow the instructions on how to take them even if you are not experiencing nausea at the time. Once nausea causes vomiting, it becomes more difficult to control. I have received phone calls from patients who did not take the anti-nausea pills when they went home after treatment because they were feeling quite well. They felt well because they had received anti-nausea medication with the chemotherapy. The additional pills are meant to prevent delayed nausea.

Anecdotes exist about patients encountering their cancer doctor or nurse years later in an unrelated setting like a ski slope or a supermarket and becoming ill from the triggered memory! So it is best to control nausea and prevent vomiting in the first place.

Hair loss is caused by loss of hair follicles. Hair follicles are in a similar state of division and growth as cancer cells and are similarly vulnerable to chemotherapy drugs. Follicles do recover after chemotherapy, but no useful measures prevent hair loss during it. People have tried different techniques to minimize hair loss such as wearing ice caps during chemotherapy. They have been mostly unsuccessful. The FDA has approved a similar device, and it may be worth exploring. Some drugs do not cause complete hair loss, and your hair may only thin out. If total hair loss is expected, your doctor will prescribe a wig. If you get the wig before you lose your hair, the wig makers can match it to your natural hair very well. Even when I know which patients have lost their hair, I have difficulty telling the wig apart from their natural hair. Some people choose not to wear the wigs and go bare, wear hats or become creative with scarves. Fewer wig/toupee options exist for men because they are harder to match. You would expect to lose hair by the third week of chemotherapy, and it can then take from two to four months after treatment is completed for your hair to grow back to its full thickness. Hair starts growing back right away, but it will take that much time to become wig-free. The color and curl will be different, and people are often surprised by your new look.

Even if hair loss is temporary, the mention of it during the discussion of chemotherapy causes distress. It is the single visible sign of cancer and its treatment, and it brings home the emotional reality of the disease. Since other effects of the chemotherapy are not visible to you or to others, the hair loss can be an emotional trigger point. It's OK. You are not alone in that distress.

Additional side effects will depend on the drugs being used. Some cause diarrhea. Others cause tingling or numbness in the fingers or toes called neuropathy. Others cause changes in liver, kidney, or heart function, all of which will be monitored carefully with blood work for the liver and kidneys and heart scans for the heart. With vigilance we try to catch any changes before any real damage takes place

How is chemotherapy given?.

Most chemotherapy is given into a vein; the prescribed dose is mixed into a saline or glucose bag, and it enters your circulation directly. Some infusions take a few minutes, some take a few hours, and some take several days with the help of a portable pump.

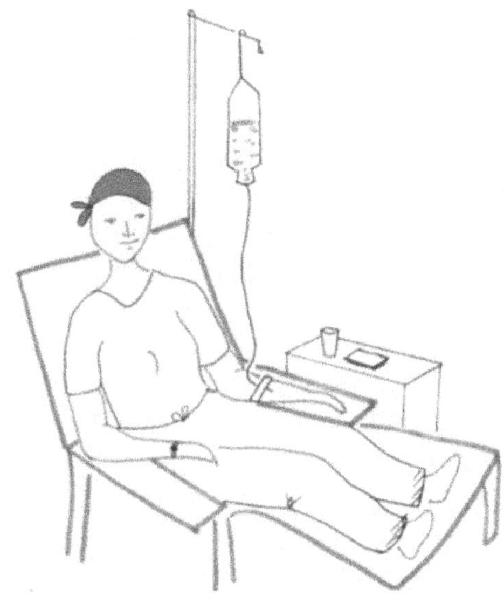

Getting intravenous chemotherapy

Figure 13.2

Does chemotherapy come in pill form? My neighbor is taking chemotherapy pills. Why do I get intravenous treatment?

Some cancers are now being treated with pills, but they are still in the minority. Most cancers still need intravenous treatment. Pills need to be taken dependably, on schedule daily or twice daily. You may need to set an alarm as a reminder.

You will still need to have blood work and take anti-nausea medications. You will still need to come in for regular checkups. Most of the newer oral medications fall into the "targeted therapy" category rather than chemotherapy. See the section on targeted therapy in Chapter 10.

Why are chemotherapy drugs given in combinations?

Different chemotherapy drugs work at different points of the cell division cycle. The combinations are usually more powerful than a single drug. In curative treatments it is necessary to be aggressive to eradicate all cancer cells.

Why are the treatments given repeatedly?

Almost all chemotherapy drugs target cells that are preparing to divide or are actually in the cell division phase. Any cells in the rest or growth phase are not vulnerable to chemotherapy. At the time of each drug infusion only some of the cancer cells are in their weak or vulnerable phase. Those cells are killed, but the rest of the cancer cells continue to grow as they progress to the preparation and division phase after the chemotherapy drugs have left the body.

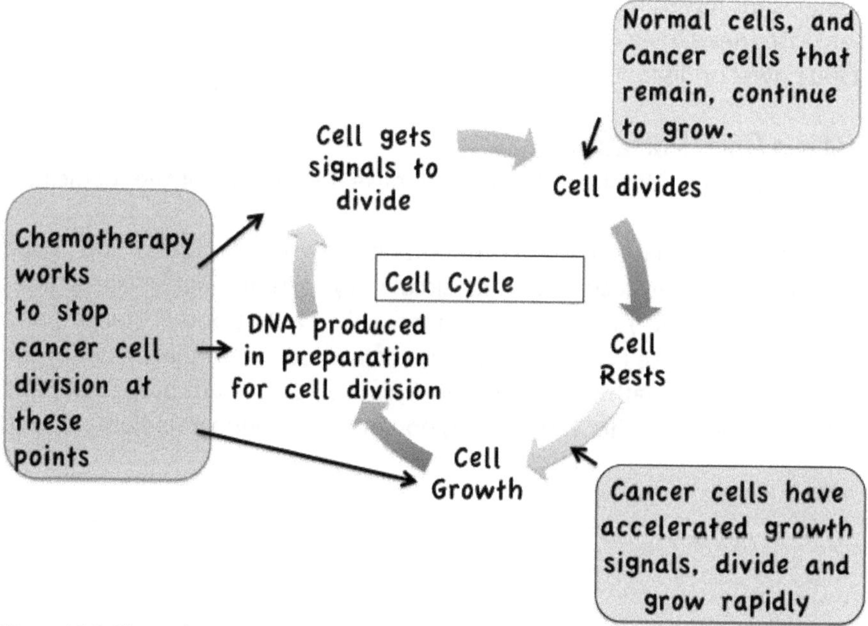

Figure 13.3 Chemotherapy targets in the Cell Cycle

We give chemotherapy in intervals to give the normal cells a chance to recover, but it needs to be given repeatedly to keep hitting the cancer cells. When my children were toddlers, they played with a game called whack-a-mole. Plastic moles popped up and down through holes in a plastic platform, and the kids whacked at them with plastic hammers. The goal was to hit as many as you could before they popped back in again. Treating cancer with chemotherapy is like whack-a-mole. Repeat cycles of chemotherapy try to get as many cancer cells as they can with each treatment. Treatments are spaced far enough apart to give the body a chance to recover but to catch the next batch of cancer cells in their weak or vulnerable phase.

Can I get too much chemotherapy?

Chemotherapy is prescribed according to a formula which takes into account your body weight and height. The formula gives us a number called the Body Surface Area (BSA), and chemotherapy doses are calculated according to your BSA. This dose will change from treatment to treatment if you gain or lose weight because this will change your BSA. In addition, your doctor may alter the dose if there are changes in your blood counts or in the way your kidneys or liver are working. Standard treatment plans have standard doses as well as guidelines for lowering the doses when necessary. Trigger points determine when doses need to be decreased by a certain percentage or treatment needs to be delayed or discontinued.

What is a Port (PortaCath)?

"I have bad veins. What can be done to make it easier to get the medicines into my blood?"

If you expect to have many treatments, it may be difficult to find "good veins." To get easier access to your circulatory system, doctors sometimes place a device inside your chest commonly called a Port or a Portacath, or a Venous Access Device (VAD). The Port is a coin-sized device placed under the skin in the area beneath the collarbone. This is an outpatient procedure, and the device is placed either by your Surgeon or Interventional Radiologist, and

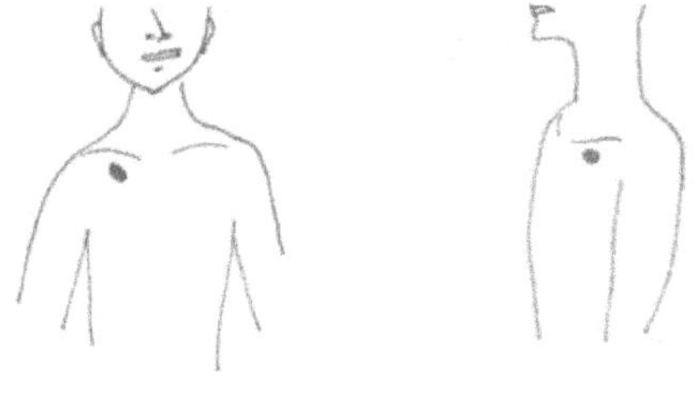

Portacath commonly placed under collar bone.

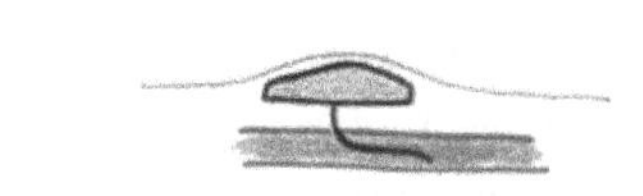

Inserted under the skin, catheter feeds into a large vein.

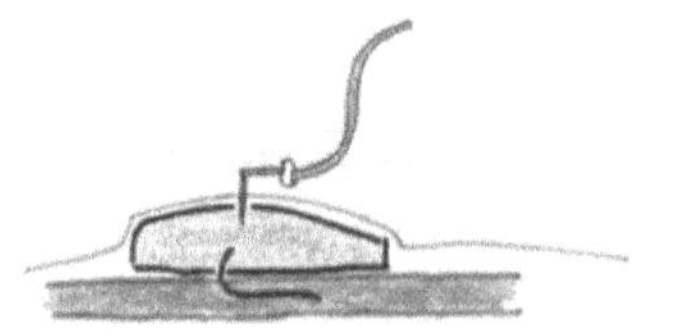

Chemotherapy infusion needle inserted into portacath when needed, removed after infusion finished.

Figure 13.4 The Portacath

it is done under local anesthesia. When the Port is not being used, there is no external catheter or needle to take care of. Most Ports are only used for chemo or intravenous fluids. Some special Powerports can be used for blood transfusions, and some multi-chamber Ports can be used for more than one type of infusion (for either antibiotics or intravenous nutrition).

I only have a few treatments. Do I really need a Port?

One of the downsides of intravenous chemotherapy is the need to get an IV line inserted into your arm each time you have an infusion. Doctors do not want to use a vein in the crook of your elbow or a thin vein on the back of your hand. We do not want the needle to slip out of your vein and the chemotherapy to leak into your skin tissue. Dehydration makes veins more difficult to access, and repeated treatments can damage smaller veins. Using a Port makes treatment easier and safer. When the treatments are completed, the device can be removed.

Can the Port be used for blood work?

Usually only a trained nurse is permitted to use the Port, because after each use a small dose of a blood thinner is put into the chamber to prevent clotting. Most outpatient labs do not have a person qualified to do this. If you can only have blood work through your Port, you must make an appointment for that in the infusion center.

Why do I get blood tests so often? I have so little to begin with.

Blood tests are necessary to measure how your body's normal cells are responding to the chemotherapy. As the chemotherapy circulates through the bone marrow, the normal blood cell production is affected. The blood test for a complete blood count (CBC) will tell us how low your counts dropped between treatments and if the marrow has recovered enough for the next treatment. If it has not, treatment may need to be delayed or doses may need to be adjusted.

Similarly, we need to make sure that your kidneys and your liver are working well enough to process the next chemotherapy treatment.

You do have enough blood in your circulation for these blood tests. In general, the blood work takes about 1-2 ml out of 5000 ml that you have, and your body replaces it fairly quickly. People can become anemic from blood tests usually only when they are hospitalized and blood tests are done at least daily, and sometimes four to six times a day, for days at a time. This is not the case for routine outpatient chemotherapy.

Can the blood tests tell if my cancer is gone?

These blood tests do not tell us whether there are any active cancer cells. Researchers are trying to develop tests that measure cancer cells in your blood stream in special situations, but they are not currently available for routine use. Such tests may become available at some point both to guide therapy and to establish whether or not you are in remission.

What will help my blood counts recover faster?

There is nothing you can eat or drink that will help your counts recover faster. The bone marrow recovers on its own timetable. Recovery slows down even further as the treatment continues. If low blood counts delay treatment repeatedly, doses can be adjusted to minimize the effect. We try to avoid dose reduction in curative treatments because the chemotherapy dose is usually very specific.

However, some injections can be administered the day after chemotherapy to decrease the vulnerable period. Some injections improve the red cell count. Your treating team will decide if you need these injections and whether it is safe for you to get them.

Do I have to stay at home and avoid visitors when I get Chemotherapy?

No, you do not have to stay at home for the most part. The vulnerable periods for infection are mid cycle when the white count is the lowest. You will know this through your blood work. Mid-cycle tests are routinely performed only with the first cycle, but they can be added at any time you report feeling excessively tired or have a fever. During this vulnerable period, visitors who are sick should not visit. You may also want to wear a mask over your nose and mouth for precaution. It is wise to avoid closed and crowded spaces like movie theatres or crowded public transportation, especially during flu season. If you have the ability to work from home, or telecommute, you could use that option. Keep up with your flu vaccinations. Your chemotherapy treatments do not affect your ability to develop immunity to the flu, and the vaccination will protect you.

And always use good hand hygiene. Wash your hands frequently and use hand sanitizers.

Can I work during chemotherapy?

It depends on the nature of your job and the nature of your chemotherapy. If your job will not allow flexible hours or days off when needed, for example manufacturing or service industry jobs, you may need to take medical leave. If your job requires travelling, you may not be able to continue working because chemotherapy schedules are reasonably rigid, and you may be suffering from fatigue or other side effects for a few days after each treatment. If your job allows you to work from home, many patients do prefer to continue working a reduced schedule. Some people, however, are only slightly affected by side effects and are able to continue all their activities.

We cannot really predict who will sail through chemotherapy and who will not. If you have already lost weight, or if your digestive tract or lungs are affected, you may need to take time off. If your treatment is a preventive treatment, and you are not debilitated, you may be able to carry on quite well. Every patient is different. You will find out when you go through treatment.

How many treatments do I need?

If your treatment is curative, a standard number of treatments is required to get rid of the cancer cells. The number depends on the disease and stage. They range from four to twelve treatments given at regular intervals and are on a fairly strict schedule. The chemotherapy drugs need to keep hitting the cancer cells that are entering the vulnerable phase, and the intervals are scheduled to do so.

If the treatment is palliative, it is designed to decrease and control the size of the tumors, not to eradicate them. The treatment is ongoing and the end point is open-ended. Since the cancer cells are still present at any point, stopping the chemotherapy will allow them to grow again. Treatment breaks are possible, however, and are built into the plan. Dose and schedule adjustments can be made to make the treatment a bit easier for the long term.

We will talk more about curative and palliative treatments in Chapter 14 where we will discuss the goals of treatment.

Can I exercise when I am undergoing chemotherapy?

You should exercise as much as you can tolerate. Going through cancer treatment is no reason to give up on exercise. Now is the time to continue moderate and appropriate exercise. Obviously it needs to be modified depending on any surgery you have undergone. Abdominal crunches would not be appropriate after an abdominal operation, and using a weight bench would not be appropriate after a breast operation.

Walking is the best exercise during treatment. Walk at as brisk a pace as you can manage for 15-20 minutes daily. Walk more if you can manage it. Fifteen repetitions of biceps curls with two to five pound hand weights and climbing up and down a flight of stairs three or four times daily will keep you in good condition. After your treatment ends, you can pick up the pace and intensity.

For some patients treatments will not end for a long time. Consulting with a physical therapist about how much they can and should do is important.

Doctors used to think that exercise after breast cancer surgery was harmful. That has been disproven. In fact, light to moderate exercise has been shown to be beneficial in maintaining conditioning, mobility, and a sense of well-being. After treatments are finished, it is important to keep up with an exercise routine and maintain a healthy weight.

Alan lost much of his conditioning during his multiple surgeries, and he became unable to do anything for himself. We recommended physical therapy in his home. The therapists started working with him twice a week, and his mobility and endurance improved significantly. It made him much more independent.

What is chemo brain?

Patients undergoing chemotherapy often complain that their brain feels "foggy." They cannot process information or think at their usual levels. Often this fogginess lasts for a few months, and recovery can take up to a year. Previously doctors did not understand that this was a real "brain-related" condition. They believed that most chemotherapy drugs were prevented from entering the brain by a functional barrier called the "blood-brain barrier." Women have complained about these symptoms for decades (men experienced them as well), but the symptoms were often attributed to depression, fatigue, poor nutrition, and lack of exercise.

Recent studies, however, have validated this phenomenon of chemo-brain. Eventually we will get data about recovery time and extent of recovery. Exercise has been shown to decrease the effects of chemo brain.

Do I have to stay in the hospital for chemotherapy?

Very few treatment plans require hospitalization. Most treatment is now delivered as an outpatient. Some treatments take a few minutes and some take a few hours. If a 24-hour infusion is required, and it is safe to do so, it can be given via a portable infusion pump. You can carry this pump in a small satchel or waist pack. Your pump is loaded with the medicine and connected and disconnected in the Infusion Center.

The treatments for acute leukemia and aggressive Lymphomas do need hospitalization. You are too sick to be outside the hospital, the schedule of drugs is complicated, and side effects need more intensive management.

Why is my chemotherapy not ready when I have the appointment?

Chemotherapy is custom mixed according to your body weight and height and the results of your current blood work. If you cannot receive the treatment that day for any reason, your drugs, once mixed, cannot be used for someone else and are wasted. Doses and schedules can change because of weight loss, unexpected infections, transportation issues, weather issues, etc. After you are seen and cleared for chemotherapy, the pharmacist will prepare your treatment. This process takes time, and you will need some patience. A lot goes on behind the scenes.

If my cancer returns, can I be treated again?

Yes, you can be treated for recurrences. Unlike radiation therapy, chemotherapy can be used again. The drugs can be chosen to avoid worsening any side effects lingering from previous treatments. For example, if the previous treatment caused nerve damage, the next drug of choice would be a nerve-sparing drug if possible. Some drugs have a lifetime total dose limit, but alternate drugs can be used.

Chemotherapy Teaching Session

After your doctors finalize the treatment of choice, and if you are going to get chemotherapy, you will be scheduled for a chemotherapy teaching session. Usually a specialized Oncology Nurse or Nurse Practitioner will give you a detailed description of the drugs, their side effects, and instructions about what to do to prevent or treat symptoms resulting from their use. Prescriptions for anti-nausea medications and any other supportive services that may be required are prepared at this time. You will receive phone numbers for after-hours access and instructions about which situations necessitate a call to your support services.

The whole session can be overwhelming. Do attend it with someone who can listen with you and take notes. The information packet can seem excessively detailed, so ask for the key points to remember. Sometimes the important facts can get lost in the avalanche of information.

It is also very important to tell your Oncologist about all the over-the-counter medicines you are taking including herbal medicines and dietary supplements, because some of them may interfere with the chemotherapy treatment. Grapefruit juice, for example, can change the absorption of some oral medicines.

Neal is scheduled for a chemotherapy teaching session. Mona is going with him, and they carry the folder in which they are taking notes and a recording device in case they need to record any instructions.

After your Chemotherapy Teaching session:

You will be asked to sign a consent form for your chemotherapy treatment. You will receive your appointment for your first treatment. In some cancer centers, the teaching session and consent for treatment occur on the same day as the first treatment. In other centers it is scheduled before the first treatment.

The journey begins...

Neal finishes his chemotherapy teaching session and is scheduled for his Port placement. He will pick up his anti-nausea medicines from his pharmacy before the treatment starts. He is going to have chemotherapy once a week and radiation every day for six or seven weeks. He receives a calendar that will remind him of his daily schedule. The two teams (radiation and chemotherapy) will be in touch with each other about his progress.

New members of your team

- Oncology Nurse Practitioner
- Chemotherapy Infusion Nurse
- Radiation Therapist
- Pharmacist
- Social Worker
- Dietician
- Physical Therapist
- Financial Counselor

Things to take care of...

- Dental care if you need it.
- Check if you need to be on Short Term Disability during treatment.
- Transportation arrangements.
- Family medical leave papers if your family is going to take time off from work.
- Get your flu shot if it is the flu season.
- Get a thermometer.
- Fill your prescriptions. Check into a mail order pharmacy for repeat prescriptions.
- Start or maintain an appropriate exercise routine.

Special Action Plan for Chemotherapy Teaching Session

- Take someone with you for the chemotherapy teaching session.
- Ask to record the session so you can review it again.
- Get the prescriptions you need for anti-nausea medications.
- Order a wig.
- Ask about a Port.
- Ask about Nutrition Counseling.
- Ask about Infection Precautions and Physical Activity.

Glossary:

- **Port/ Portacath/VAD**: A device placed inside your chest for intravenous infusion.
- **Infusion**: Medicine mixed into a solution and put into your blood stream via a needle inserted into your vein.
- **CBC**: A blood count measuring your white cells, which fight infection, red cells, which carry hemoglobin, and platelet cells, which are needed to stop bleeding.

14. Defining The Goals Of Your Treatment

Neal attends the planning sessions for radiation and chemotherapy. As he listens to the potential complications of treatment and how difficult it is going to be, he wonders if this is worth it.

How will this Treatment help me?

This is an important question both to ask and to answer as you make decisions with your doctor about your cancer treatment.

When you are first diagnosed, you do not want to lose any more time than necessary. You have already waited for the biopsy results, attended the consultations, and had the scans required for staging. Now you want to get started on the treatment. We are surrounded by a culture of "fight the cancer." Patients do not commonly ask whether, or how much, the treatment will help them. It is normal to be afraid of answers you may not want to hear.

Addressing these issues in the beginning, however, helps to be more informed and more prepared for what the future may hold. You and your doctor can then make treatment decisions according to your life goals.

What are treatment decisions based on?

Treatment is tailored to the...

Stage of cancer: Can this cancer be cured or not? If the goal is cure, then strong treatment may be necessary. If the cancer is advanced, the treatment is palliative and will be milder for reasons that we will discuss further in this chapter.

Nature of the cancer: Is the cancer cell aggressive and fast growing? If the answer is yes, the risk of relapse is higher, and you might select stronger treatment. If the cell is a low-grade cell, a milder treatment may be sufficient for success. We described assessing the future behavior of the cancer cell in Chapter 5 on interpreting the pathology report.

Performance Status: This standardized measurement of your functional abilities (ADLs or activities of daily living) is linked to your ability to withstand treatment and your strength and ability to carry out daily tasks. Are you up and about most of the day? Can you wash, dress, and feed yourself? Are you in pain? Do your symptoms limit your physical abilities? The weaker you are to begin with, the less likely you are to get through treatment without difficulty. If you can climb a flight of stairs, go to work, and do all your ADLs, you have a good performance status. As your physical abilities worsen, your performance status goes down. This measures increasing weakness and predicts difficulty for tolerating continued treatments.

Other illnesses: Kidney failure, cardiac disease, badly controlled diabetes, neuropathy, and other chronic conditions all affect your ability to withstand strong treatment. All treatments have side effects and can make existing conditions worse. Existing illnesses require active management in a team approach with your other specialists.

Age: Age is an indirect gauge of health. Older people often have other illnesses such as congestive heart failure. They may be more frail. If the cancer is slow growing, their life expectancy may be related to their age and other medical conditions rather than to their cancer. They may be better off with observation alone. Slow growing prostate cancer in older men is a good example. If an older patient has a good performance status and no other major medical conditions, age is not a barrier to standard curative treatment.

What is curative treatment?

Curative treatment can eliminate all evidence of cancer with an expectation of long-term disease-free survival. In most cancers it is limited to Stage 1 through Stage 3 with the best results being for Stage 1. Curative treatment plans can include any of the methods of treatment described in Chapter 10. It may be surgery alone or surgery followed by a prescribed number of chemotherapy treatments or a series of chemotherapy treatments alone. It depends on the type of cancer and the stage. Even if the treatment is strong, once it ends, you can recover from the side effects.

Why is Stage 4 cancer not curable?

If the cancer has spread to distant organs like the brain, bones, liver, or lungs, it cannot be eradicated or cured. This spread of cancer cells to secondary sites is called metastases, and aggressive treatment for the primary or even the visible secondary sites will not eradicate or cure all disease. There are cancer cells in transit which will create new secondary sites when they lodge in a new place. Treatment is designed for disease control.

Then what is remission?

Remission is the absence of visible disease after treatment. Some diseases are known to "disappear" after treatment but "reappear" months or even years later. Some low-grade Lymphomas disappear with treatment, but they relapse in time and require another round of treatment.

Are some Stage 4 cancers curable?

There are a few current exceptions to the "no cure" rule.

Testicular cancer: Lance Armstrong is an elite cyclist who was diagnosed with metastatic cancer that had spread to his brain. He was successfully treated and cured of his disease and went on to compete in tough cycling races.

Blood and lymph node related cancers, for example Stage 4 lymphomas and leukemia, a cancer of the cells of the bone marrow, have a chance to be eradicated with aggressive chemotherapy.

This is a short list, but it will change in the future as researchers make advances in treatments. Some targeted Immunotherapy is showing very promising results in melanoma as we saw with President Jimmy Carter. After four months of taking treatment, his brain metastases seem to have disappeared.

What is palliative care?

Palliative care addresses both the effects of the cancer and the side effects of its treatment. Even if the disease has spread outside the primary organ, treatment can often still be helpful in extending life by slowing the growth of the Cancer.

Tumors cause symptoms by their physical presence because they occupy space in a confined area pushing aside normal structures and invading nerves and blood vessels. This can cause pain and swelling, and shrinking the tumors can help relieve those symptoms. Tumors decrease the amount of functioning normal tissue and cause decreased organ function. Loss of functioning lung tissue can cause breathing difficulty, or blocked airways can cause pneumonias.

Tumors can block ducts or passages. If the duct along which urine flows from the kidney to the bladder is blocked, a stent, or tube, can be placed inside that duct to keep it open. This can allow the urine to continue to flow and decrease possible loss of kidney function. Stents can also be placed in the bile duct and other passages that are obstructed such as the esophagus (food pipe) or the rectum. Placing such tubes often avoids the need for surgery.

Treatment often causes side effects and can make the patient very weak. Depression can be debilitating and decrease motivation to take care of yourself. Poor nutrition can worsen weight loss.

Combinations of different medications can better control pain, nausea, constipation, weight loss, anxiety, depression, and other symptoms caused by the cancer and its treatment. Physical therapy can improve conditioning, mobility, and balance and reduce the risk of falls.

By treating these symptoms, doctors can improve the quality of life.

Why is non-curative or palliative treatment milder? Shouldn't we be using stronger treatment because the cancer has spread?

Since the cancer cannot be eradicated, treatment is usually planned for an unlimited number of cycles. It often continues until the tumors start growing bigger. When this happens a different treatment is offered if the patient's physical condition will allow it. The new treatment plan will take into account any weakness or organ damage which can make it difficult for the patient to tolerate more treatment.

Since palliative chemotherapy treatment is indefinite, it is purposely milder to minimize the buildup of side effects. Ongoing chemotherapy, therefore, needs to be tailored to the patient's wishes, life expectancy, performance status, and life goals.

There are tradeoffs to this choice.

Treatment causes side effects which can be mild or severe. Fatigue, infections, dehydration, anemia, blood transfusion, and hospitalizations may be the price to pay for ongoing treatment. An honest discussion is necessary to make the right choice. That extra time may get you to your grandchild's graduation and may be worthwhile to you. Or you may decide that the side effects impact badly on your quality of life, and the possibility of the extra weeks or months is not worth it to you. Many patients think they have to keep getting treatment because they don't want to disappoint their family. You are not letting anyone down. It's OK to decide to stop treatment.

Questions to consider...

Is it worth going through treatment if I can't be cured?

Define your treatment goals. Some people may want to live until a daughter graduates from high school or college or gets married. Others may want to finish a project, take a planned trip, make peace with their loved ones, or enjoy the summer. How far away is that target? Make sure that the recommended treatment can let you achieve your goals. If it cannot, try to move the target. When I have a conversation about treatment goals with my patients, I make those suggestions. Graduation dates cannot be moved, but trips or wedding dates can be rescheduled and celebrated earlier. Chemotherapy schedules can be adjusted to accommodate your needs to participate in particular events and achieve your life goals.

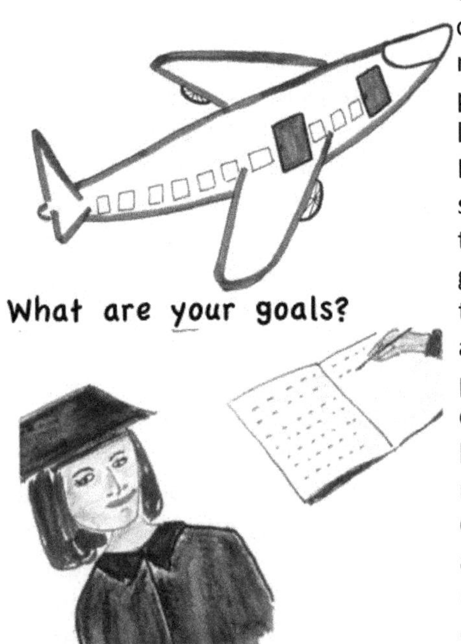

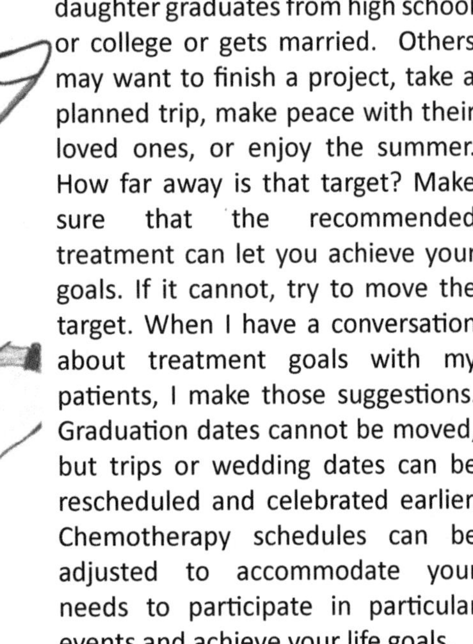

Figure 14.1

Is the treatment going to make me live longer or make my life better?

If the answer to both those questions is no, you may want to evaluate your decision carefully. If you decide that treatment is going to worsen your quality of life, you may prefer not to spend what time you have in the treatment center or in the hospital.

On the other hand, you may be at the stage in life where every additional day is critical. One of my patients lived in this pre-terminal stage for many months. The extra time enabled him to spend time with his young children and organize his finances to help take care of their future needs.

Without an honest discussion about these issues, you cannot make educated choices. A study published in the *Journal of Clinical Oncology* reported that having these discussions did not worsen sadness or anxiety. It did enable people to make realistic decisions.

It may seem early to start thinking about appointing a health care proxy and deciding what life support measures you might want. Most people, both physicians and patients, put off this discussion until a crisis forces them to decide. Having this discussion in the middle of a crisis often leads to poor decisions. Introducing the topic when discussing treatment goals makes it routine and normal. Patients have a chance to truly think about and communicate their wishes to their family and physician. Making a decision one way initially is not irrevocable. You can change your mind as your treatment proceeds.

If you decide against pursuing active cancer treatment in any form, we will address options for care and comfort and hospice care in Chapter 24.

Do I have to start treatment immediately?

Only cancers that are very rapidly growing, like acute leukemia (a cancer of the bone marrow), need to be treated urgently. Most other kinds of cancers do not grow dangerously fast and need to be fully staged before starting treatment. There is time to consider all your options before making a decision.

Is it worthwhile to enroll in a clinical trial?

We will address that question in the chapter on Clinical Trials (Chapter 19). At this stage, while you are evaluating your goals of treatment, it will depend on your disease, whether you are newly diagnosed, or whether the disease has grown in spite of treatment.

What is a Health Care Proxy (HCP)?

A HCP is a person you designate to make medical decision on your behalf if you are incapacitated and unable to make your own decisions. It can be your spouse, partners, adult child, trusted friend, lawyer, or anyone you choose to designate.

What are Advance Directives?

Advance Directives are instructions you give in advance about many medical questions. Do you want cardiac resuscitation, a breathing machine, or artificial nutrition by stomach tube? A form called the MOLST form, or Medical Orders for Life Sustaining Treatment, addresses these questions. Signing such a form provides instructions about what interventions you do or do not wish.

You can obtain the MOLST form from your doctor's office, and there is a sample copy in the appendix.

Neal decides that even if the treatment is harsh, he has a fighting chance of a cure. He wants more time with his wife and family. He wants to see his grandchildren grow up. He decides that he will proceed with treatment. Although his family is wary of the toll the treatment will take on Neal, they are very happy and supportive of his choice.

Questions to ask:

- Is my treatment curative? When can we start? Is it critical to start right away?
- If my treatment will not be curative, is it necessary to start right away?
- Will this treatment extend my life? By how much? What are the side effects?
- What are my other options?
- Will I benefit from a clinical trial?

Action Plan

- Know the stage of your disease.
- Review the success rate of the recommended treatment.
- Decide if the benefits of the treatment are in keeping with your life expectancy.

Section D

What else can help you?

"In God we trust. All others [must] have data."

Bernard Fisher, M.D.
Oncologist, Researcher.

15. How to Deal with Advice?

Neal starts his treatment. He and Mona get a lot of advice on how to fight his cancer, which doctors to see, where to get treated, what to eat, what not to eat, and how to keep his immune system active. Someone wants him to try some herbs that their aunt took. Another friend looks up the "best place" for his cancer to be treated and urges Neal to go there. Sound familiar?

Advice: Help or Hindrance?

How do you deal with advice?

Advice from well meaning friends and relatives is a double-edged sword. Depending on your situation, and who is giving the advice, it can be helpful, cumbersome, or distinctly unhelpful.

Let us make sure you have enough refills on your nausea medicine. Shall I go to the Pharmacy for you?

Helpful Advice: Friends and relatives do mean well, and advice can certainly be helpful. Friends or relatives may have personal or professional experience with your situation and be able to guide you through the process much like this book will. They can help you anticipate and deal with situations as they arise. Through the years many friends and relatives have asked me for advice. I have offered any help they may need in understanding their condition, but I have been careful not to give advice if it is not requested.

Cumbersome advice: People can be relentless in suggesting you try various treatments, or dietary or naturopathic treatment, which may not be helpful to your situation. A number of my patients have been confused by the advice that is thrown at them: Drink this; Don't eat that; Try this special tea that boosts your immunity; My aunt had this treatment and did horribly. That sort of advice is not helpful because it does not offer encouragement and support and can conflict with what medical information actually says.

My neighbor said you must drink this drink. His wife also gave up root vegetables. And sugar. And dairy.

Unhelpful advice: People can provide misinformation which may not be relevant to your situation. It is particularly disturbing if the bad information sends you into a state of unnecessary panic.

My aunt was in the ICU for weeks after her surgery. It went very badly for her. I'm not sure if you should do this.

Here is an example of misinformation.

My friend called me to say that her neighbor, Nina, was in need of some urgent advice. Nina's 17-year-old son had been diagnosed with a brain tumor. One night she arrived at my friend's house in a panic. Someone had dropped off information about a particular variety of brain cancer that has a bad outcome. Luckily for her I was able to look at that information and reassure her that her son had the kind of tumor that was not aggressive. Her son's expected outcome was quite good given the correct treatment. Not everyone has a neighbor who has an oncologist friend, so you need to find a way of handling all volunteer advice. You could respond by saying that you don't have all your reports yet and you understand that everyone's cancer is different.

What to do with advice to use supplements?

"My cousin brought me these pills; she says they are "natural" and will help my body fight the cancer. Can I take them?" A lot of advice from friends and relatives is about taking vitamins and supplements.

Many years ago anti-oxidant pills were very popular. They contained extra doses of Vitamin E and C and minerals. Research later noted that excess Vitamin E actually correlated with a poorer treatment outcome and could even cause complications.

This is not to say some supplements may not have some benefit, but do your own research to see if any scientific studies support such claims. Anecdotes do not count as evidence. Consult Chapter 17 for more information on supplements and complementary and alternative treatments.

Most importantly, ask your medical team. I always ask my patients what supplements they are taking in addition to their prescription medications. That list is often quite long. Doctors want to make sure any supplements you take will not interfere with your recommended treatment.

What can you do with bad information?

How can you determine which information is bad or unreliable? You will need to judge both where that information originated and your relationship with the giver. You need to consult your medical team if you need clarification.

You may need a practiced response, and your response may depend on where you are in your treatment. You might prepare a folder where you file all suggestions without reading anything until after you have your consultations. You might hand it back, saying, " Can you hold it for me until I see my Oncologist? I don't want to read the bad part yet." Or you could say, "Thank you, but I am waiting to do my research until after I get all my reports so I know I am researching the correct condition." Even though the others mean well, you can still call the shots.

How to take help?

People don't know what you need, but they would like to help. Do take offered help. You could need help with chores or errands or rides to treatment or to the pharmacy to pick up medications. Having a meal dropped off might be wonderful. If your children or parents need your help, your friend could help with their needs and thus help you. Sometimes it is simply nice to have someone drop by for company. A number of different offers can be useful. Psychologically it helps to know you have a community with you.

If you are savvy with online calendars, you can set up a calendar where people can sign up to give you rides or deliver meals. Or one of your helpful friends can set it up for you.

If you are a friend or relative reading this, try not to share all your "bad outcome" anecdotes. That is not helpful. For reasons that are not clear, it is fairly common to narrate all the bad stories instead of the good ones. "My aunt had that treatment, and she had such bad vomiting that she had to be hospitalized after every treatment." "My neighbor had an allergic reaction to the CT scan dye and almost died." The old adage holds true: If you can't say anything good (or helpful), do not say it. Every patient is different.

What you *can* do is offer support. Make meals for the family, shop for groceries, help with cleaning or picking up the kids from school. Leave the medical opinions and decisions to the patients and their doctors.

Neal and Mona have been fortunate. Their friends have offered help and buoy Neal's spirits as he faces the next few months of treatment. Friends plan to give Neal rides to the Radiation Center to give Mona a break. They visit, bring meals, and keep both Neal and Mona company.

Action Plan:

- Take advice from your Medical Professionals.
- Develop a response to other kinds of advice.
- Take help from friends and relatives.

16. What is the Role of Nutrition and Exercise?

Neal has lost weight since he started feeling ill. Now he has to work on gaining it back and preparing his body for the treatment to come.

Nutrition is always a big source of concern, both at the beginning and during the course of treatment. You may have lost weight already because of the cancer, and the doctors are telling you not to lose more weight. You need your strength to get through the treatments. Even if you have not lost weight, you need to focus on good nutrition. If you begin treatment with a healthy weight, it helps to achieve a better outcome with fewer hospital stays and better survival.

Why does cancer cause weight loss?

Reasons for weight loss caused by cancer can be varied.

- The cancer cell itself produces chemicals that suppress appetite.
- Food doesn't taste right, or you can't finish your meal.
- Tumors may be pressing on some element of your digestive tract making it difficult to eat and drink adequately. If your swallowing mechanism is not functioning properly, as happens in throat cancers, you may have fear of choking.
- You may be experiencing nausea and are afraid to eat. Chemotherapy can also change your taste for foods. Anti-nausea medicine before a meal may help, or you may wish to eat only what agrees with you.
- You may be constipated and feel full.
- Pain medications and pain itself can prevent you from feeling like eating.

- Your sense of smell may be more sensitive and make some foods unwelcome.
- Radiation therapy to the head and neck can dry up the salivary glands and cause local discomfort. It can also change how foods taste and make favorite foods unappetizing.

All this will eventually return to normal after the treatments are completed, but it can take some time. Do not get discouraged.

How do you catch up? How do you eat when you are not hungry?

"I'm not hungry. I pick at my breakfast, and I can't really eat any lunch or dinner."

Track what you eat: First of all, keep a diary of your intake. This will help track what you are actually eating (not what you think you are eating) and when. You may find that you are hungriest for breakfast or lunch rather than dinner, so make that meal count. You may not be able to eat big meals.

Supplement your meals: Add calories and protein with smoothies and shakes with added protein powder. These are available in many different flavors commercially, or you can make your own.

Choose high protein, high calorie foods: Eat peanut butter, avocados, tofu, and cream cheese, which pack a punch in a small volume and do not fill you up. Eat easily digestible lean meats and fish.

Eat frequently: Small, frequent meals are better than three meals you cannot finish. If you can only eat small quantities at a time, eat more than three meals a day.

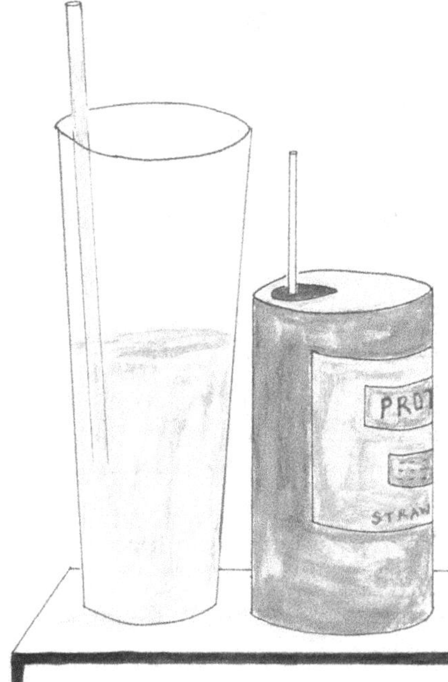

Figure 16.1

How to get your hydration?

Broths will fill you up and contribute to hydration, but they usually contain a lot of salt and do not have enough nutritional content. Drink fluids between meals, not with them, so they don't fill you up. Hydration is important, but it is better to hydrate with water than broth or juices which can contain too much sugar and salt.

Have a target of fluid intake. Two liters, or approximately eight eight-ounce glasses are recommended, but do check in with your medical team. You may need more or less fluid depending on your individual situation. If you have congestive heart failure or kidney disease, your team may limit how much liquid you are allowed to consume.

Hydrate with non-caffeinated drinks. If you develop diarrhea, it will cause dehydration, and your fluid intake will need to be increased, preferably with electrolyte solutions. How much is enough? If your mouth feels dry, you need to drink more.

Throughout your treatment and beyond, adequate and balanced nutrition and hydration are important. If you start out with a few extra pounds, you may have a small margin to weather the weight loss. But excessive weight loss (more than 10%) during cancer treatment may indicate malnutrition. Malnutrition causes medical problems, so it is important to keep a balanced, healthful diet and maintain a healthful weight.

Feed the cancer. Starve the cancer. This diet or that diet will help you fight the cancer. What should you do?

Friends and family may offer varying advice about how you should maintain your nutrition. A nutrition specialist may be helpful for guidance.

What kind of diet should I follow?

No one particular diet increases or decreases cancer cure rates. Eating one food group at the expense of the others may cause an imbalance in your nutritional intake. You need adequate protein intake so your body will not break down its own vital protein.

A balanced diet is important. A macrobiotic diet, which is high in complex carbohydrates and is plant based, may contribute to harmful weight loss because of its restrictive nature. A low sugar diet may starve the cancer cell, but you may not get adequate calories to maintain your weight.

Does sugar feed the cancer?

Cancer cells do use more glucose than normal cells, and they have mechanisms for selectively using sugar to fuel their growth. It is difficult to eliminate all sugar because normal cells need sugars for routine energy needs. The best advice is to limit your processed sugar intake and get most of your calories from protein and "good fats" like olive oil and unsaturated fats. In addition, excess sugar causes weight gain, and weight gain is bad for cancer recurrence and other diseases like heart disease.

Processed foods have many grams of hidden sugars. Be watchful about sugars hidden in most canned and bottled foods, pasta sauces, and salad dressings. As far as possible, it is better to eat less processed foods.

Registered Dieticians recommend no more than six teaspoons of sugar daily for women and nine teaspoons daily for men. They prefer natural sources of sweetness such as honey, maple syrup, and agave to processed sugar, but even those natural sugars count towards your total calories. Eat fresh fruit to satisfy your craving for sweet foods rather than pastries. Think of this sequence: Eat apples first; Eat applesauce if you can't eat a fresh apple; Have apple pie sparingly or not at all.

Special Considerations:

* **Diabetic** patients need to watch their sugar intake because their blood sugars will fluctuate with their food intake.

* **Cardiac** patients will continue to follow their low sodium guidelines. Patients who have to watch their cholesterol intake, however, can relax during treatment because the need for nutrition may trump the need for low cholesterol.

Can I drink alcohol while I am on treatment?

Doctors prefer that you limit your alcohol intake. Alcohol can make you dehydrated and can upset your stomach. Regular and high alcohol consumption can interfere with blood cell production that is necessary to replace the cells killed by chemotherapy. Pain medications in combination with alcohol can change your reflexes excessively and slow you down. If you are at a wedding or another celebration, however, you may be able to join in the toast!

What food safety precautions should I take?

When you are on chemotherapy, your immunity is low, and you have to watch for food borne illnesses. Follow general food safety rules.

- Wash your hands well with soap and warm water before any food preparation.
- Keep meat, fish, and produce separate from each other.

- Refrigerate food promptly after buying.
- Do not thaw food on the kitchen counter; thaw it in the refrigerator or microwave or in cold water. Use thawed food promptly.
- Check cans to make sure they are not dented. Dented or damaged cans can harbor bacteria.
- Buy pasteurized milk and milk products.
- Cook meat and fish well. Use meat thermometers.
- Cook eggs until yolks and whites are firm.
- Boil soups and gravy when reheating.
- Reheat deli meats and hot dogs.
- Wash all salad ingredients well.
- Cook all vegetables.

Overcoming specific issues.

Smells: The smell of food being cooked can be bothersome. Ask the cook to keep the kitchen door closed while cooking, or buy more takeout than usual. Cold or room temperature foods have less odor than hot foods. Try drinking supplements through a straw to keep the drink further away from your nose.

Nausea can be minimized with small, frequent meals or starchy foods like crackers, rice or noodles, cold food or bland food. Avoid greasy, fried, or rich foods.

Diarrhea requires constant rehydration. Drink a cup of water, sports drinks, broth, or diluted juice after each loose stool, or suck on a popsicle. Bland and easy-to-digest foods like bananas, rice, applesauce and toast (the BRAT diet), or pasta are helpful. Limit dairy because lactose may aggravate diarrhea. Avoid fried or spicy foods. Your oncologist's office will give you instructions about taking medications for diarrhea and advise you when you need to call if it's not controlled. You may need intravenous hydration.

Mouth sores or difficulty swallowing will require soft foods like mashed potatoes, cream soups, custards, or pureed foods. Avoid acidic or salty food or drink such as citric or tomato-based foods.

Sense of taste can be affected by chemotherapy, other medications, or radiation therapy to the mouth. You may need to experiment with different flavors and temperatures of foods. Stronger flavors may work better than bland ones. You may have a metallic taste in your mouth. Try a baking soda rinse: a pinch of salt and baking soda in warm water. Keep a jug handy, and use this several times a day to wash out your mouth.

Speech and swallowing evaluation and therapy will help identify specific problems with the swallowing process. If swallowing is a problem, food can go down the wrong passage and enter the airways which can cause pneumonia. The speech and swallowing therapist will teach you which foods and consistencies will go down more easily. Pureed foods or thickened liquids may be easier to swallow. Swallowing exercises and chin position will help the food go down the correct passage.

What if I really can't consume the calories to regain the weight that I need?

Some cancers that involve the gastrointestinal tract or throat may make it physically very difficult to keep up with the calorie requirements. There are alternatives to eating by mouth. If there is a physical obstruction to swallowing, a tube can be placed directly into the stomach that will deliver liquid nutrition directly into the stomach, bypassing the throat, and avoiding malnourishment and dehydration during treatment. It is usually temporary and does not interfere with any food or drink that can be swallowed.

If your digestive system cannot handle liquid food via a feeding tube, special nutrition solutions can be infused directly into the blood stream. This is called Total Parenteral Nutrition, or TPN. The infused solutions are rich in fats and glucose and contain added electrolytes and vitamins. They need to be monitored very carefully and are not a permanent solution to nutrition issues.

After treatment is over....

Once you have finished your treatments, you should strive to maintain a normal weight. Focus on a sensible low fat diet containing plenty of fruits and vegetables. Maintaining a normal BMI will decrease the risk of cancer relapse. Studies have shown improvement in the outcome in breast, prostate, and colon cancers when the patient's BMI is normal.

What is BMI?

The body mass index is a value calculated from the weight (in kilograms) and height in (meters) and is expressed as kg/ m2.

The commonly accepted BMI ranges are

Underweight	Under 18.5
Normal Weight	18.5-25
Overweight	25-30
Obese	Over 30

Exercise is recommended both during and after completing cancer treatments.

"But I'm so tired. All I want to do is lie on the sofa and take a nap."

We used to tell patients to take it easy, but studies have established that keeping active through exercise helps reduce fatigue while you are going through treatments.

Exercise helps with cardiovascular endurance. Your heart is a muscle, and keeping active will help maintain good function. Exercise also induces deep breathing which will improve lung function.

Exercise generally helps with muscle conditioning, builds endurance, and helps with improving mood and self-esteem during treatment. It also helps you sleep better at night, but be sure not to exercise right before bedtime. Exercise then may energize not relax you!

What kinds of exercise can I do, and how much should I do?

Start with walking or a stationary bicycle for 10 minutes at a time. You can build up to several 10-15 minute sessions during the day. Aim for at least 30 minutes of moderate exercise a day, or 150 minutes a week. You can exercise with light weights two to three times a week to maintain your muscle strength.

Pick the time when you have the most energy to do more exercise. If you prefer company, make the exercise a social activity. If the weather is good, walking around a park is a great idea. You can rest on the park benches If you get tired, and you get some fresh air. If it's raining or snowing, or too hot and humid, and you can get to get to a mall, plan to walk in the mall. Being out and about can be uplifting for your mood.

Exercise can be any physical activity you enjoy and will stick with, for example a power walk with friends, dancing, or a zumba class. Mixing it up helps to keep it fun and uses different sets of muscles. People with arthritis can do swimming or water aerobics. The buoyancy of the water takes the pressure off painful joints.

Depending on where you live, you may be able to find special programs to build strength and endurance for cancer patients through the local hospital at their physical therapy department, the senior center, or at the local gym or YMCA. Organizations like LiveStrong have designed special programs for cancer patients and cancer survivors.

Both exercise and sensible nutrition will help maintain your BMI in a normal range. This will decrease you cancer recurrence risk.

You have put so much effort into fighting your cancer. Now stay with the program and finish the job!

Neal and Mona meet with the nutritionist before starting treatment. She provides suggestions for a meal plan and ways to supplement Neal's calories with protein rich foods or drinks when eating becomes difficult. Neal also resolves to continue his daily walk even if he has to cut it short on some days.

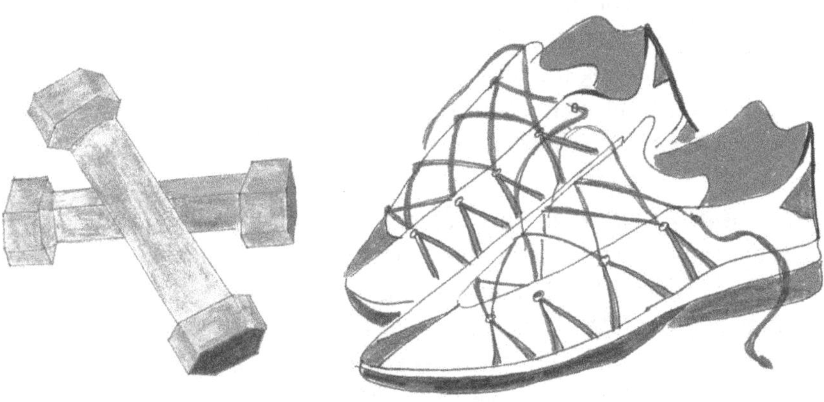

Figure 16.2 Figure 16.3

Additional resources:

- http://www.nutrition.gov/nutrition-and-health-issues/cancer
- www.aicr.org

Watch for weight gain:

Not all cancers or cancer treatments will cause weight loss. Continue moderate exercise as approved by your medical team and limit fats and sugars. Weight gain can be caused by decreased activity due to fatigue and decreased conditioning. Hormone changes that may occur because of treatments may change your metabolism. You may find yourself seeking comfort in the wrong kinds of 'comfort foods.' In the long run excess weight is a risk factor for cancer recurrence and other medical conditions.

Note: Some weight gain is related to kidney or heart failure and is caused by fluid retention.

Nutrition Action Plan:

- If you need to, consult with the dietician or speech and swallowing therapist.
- Maintain adequate nutrition and hydration.
- Clean, separate, cook, and chill your foods carefully.
- Limit alcohol and caffeinated beverages.
- Continue with good dental care to avoid tooth decay and gum disease.

Exercise Action Plan

- Consult a physical therapist if needed.
- Walk for 15 to 30 minutes daily or as much as you can during treatment.
- Try Yoga or Tai chi for gentle muscle conditioning and balance.

17. Can Complementary and Alternative Therapies Help?

Neal and Mona's neighbor, Sam, came to visit while they were weighing their treatment options. Sam's brother had been diagnosed with a blood cancer the year before, and he had declined chemotherapy. He had found a holistic center that was treating his chronic leukemia with Chinese herbal preparations. Neil and Mona looked at the literature and brought it up at their next Cancer Center appointment.

While complementary and alternative therapy are often grouped together, they are very different.

What is Complementary Therapy?

Complementary therapies are used in addition to conventional therapy.These are useful in dealing with the physical and psychological effects of cancer and the prescribed treatments. They are not recommended as the primary cancer treatment. They include Acupuncture, Massage Therapy, Reiki, Relaxation techniques, and Yoga. If your Center does not offer these services, they may be able to refer you to local practitioners. Services that are not covered by insurance may be available to cancer patients at reduced rates.

What is Acupuncture?

Acupuncture is a form of traditional Chinese medicine in which very fine needles are inserted into the skin at specific points for specific therapeutic effects. The acupuncture points lie along meridians in the body along which vital energy, or qi, is supposed to flow. The effects are not well understood, but there is some evidence that acupuncture helps relieve nausea associated with chemotherapy and radiation therapy. It also decreases the incidence of dry mouth caused by decreased saliva and helps maintain the swallowing function during head and neck cancer treatment.

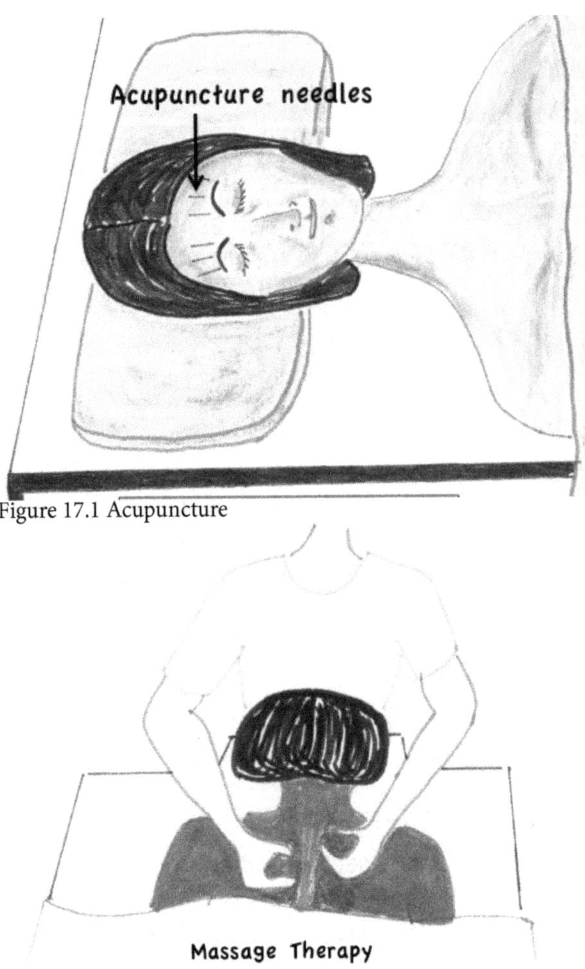

Figure 17.1 Acupuncture

Figure 17.2

What is Massage Therapy?

There are many different kinds of therapeutic massage, and many massage therapists are trained to work with cancer patients. Deep tissue massage provides pressure to deeper muscle layers to relieve chronic discomfort. Myofascial release relieves chronic myofascial syndrome. This condition causes chronic pain and inflammation of the tissue that surrounds the muscles. Trigger point massage therapy helps to relieve a tight area of a muscle which is causing pain elsewhere. Manual lymphatic drainage technique gently works and stimulates the lymphatic system to reduce localized swelling. Massage has other benefits as well. It induces relaxation, decreases heart rate, and decreases anxiety.

What is Reiki therapy?

Reiki is a form of "palm healing" or "hands on healing" developed in Japan in the early 20th century. Reiki therapists place their hands on the target area to deliver energy or heat. Especially when combined with massage, it may help relieve musculoskeletal issues. Reiki can also be used for patients who are not able to tolerate massage therapy. Cancer societies do not recommend Reiki to replace conventional treatment. Although it may be an adjunct to standard treatment, its use is not based on clinical evidence.

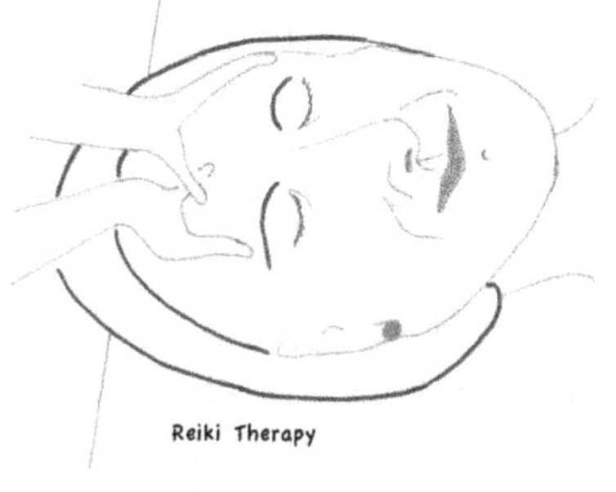

Figure 17.2 Reiki

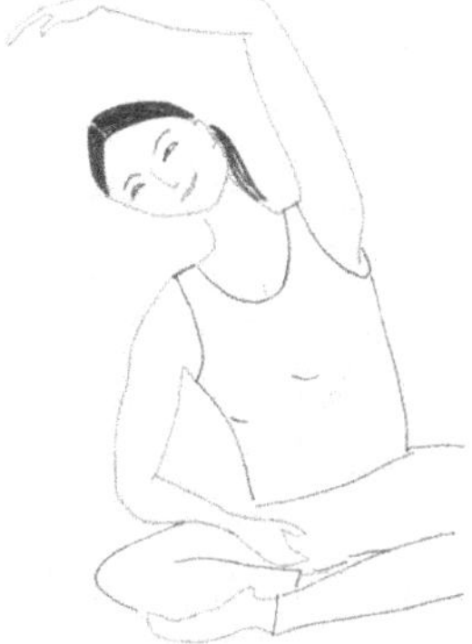

Figure 17.3 Yoga

What is Yoga?

Yoga is a spiritual, mental, and physical practice that dates back several centuries and originated in Hindu culture in India. Yoga was introduced to the Western world in the late 1800s, and the practice of yoga spread worldwide in the 20th century. As it is practiced in the West, yoga has moved away from its original Hindu spiritual roots and evolved into different schools of practice. Hatha Yoga, for example, concentrates on physical postures and breathing exercises. The poses are best learned under the guidance of a qualified yoga instructor because doing them incorrectly can cause muscle injuries.

What is Meditation?

Meditation is a spiritual practice that started thousands of years ago. Its origin is attributed to India. The practice travelled through Asia as Buddhism spread to China and Japan. In the modern era, meditation has shifted more into the realm of relaxation and self-awareness using breathing exercises, posture training, and mindfulness techniques. The practice has moved out of the religious sphere and has many health benefits. Many techniques are recommended. Commonly people assume a prescribed posture and concentrate on deep breathing. Some use a repeated word called a mantra that can help the meditator focus. Soothing sounds like recordings of the sea

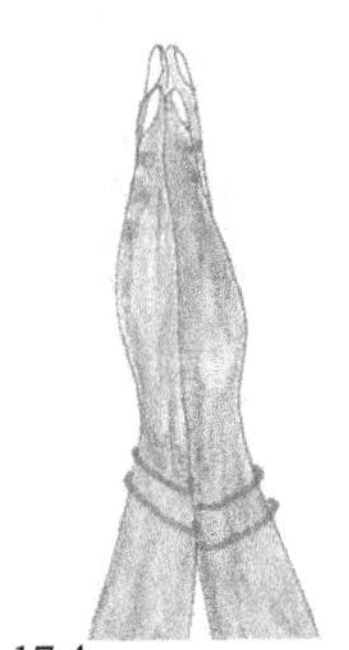
Fig. 17.4

can induce a state of relaxation.

Additional mindfulness techniques have been used to help patients deal with anxiety and addictions, pain, and chronic illnesses. All these practices can be modified to your own needs and practiced to your own satisfaction. Relaxation therapy with music, art, breathing exercises, massage, and imagery can all improve your quality of life both during and after treatment. Yoga classes are available in most cities, and meditation apps on your smartphones can help get you started.

The question of natural supplements and nutraceuticals: To take or not to take?

"Natural" supplements are very popular, and many people use them liberally to boost immunity. When patients ask me about these products, I do not have a categorical answer. In general I respond that nothing natural comes in a pill, so you should not consider these supplements to be "natural." They need to be evaluated for efficacy and safety.

What is a nutraceutical?

This sort of supplement is more accurately called a nutraceutical drug. Prescription drugs are manufactured by drug companies to deliver an active medication for a specific purpose. In order to be sold legally, pharmaceutical drugs must have their safety and efficacy established.

Nutraceuticals contain a dose of an ingredient that is naturally found in a food product. Some nutraceuticals have gone through preliminary clinical trials, have scientific backing, and have established beneficial effects. They have then suffered from lack of funding for the next phases of trials. Some nutraceuticals have been studied and used widely in countries other than the United States. Their effect may be beneficial, but they have not received FDA approval.

Some nutraceutical products have a similar, but milder, effect than their prescription counterparts because of their effect on similar pathways. Soy, for example, works on the estrogen receptor and is used to control menopausal symptoms. Red Yeast Rice helps cholesterol control as do statin drugs. Turmeric (curcumin) shows anti-inflammatory properties. It may be useful to take these in pill form because you cannot consume enough of the natural product to achieve the required medical effect. However, because they are not considered pharmaceutical drugs, nutraceuticals are sold in the dietary supplement category.

In summary, some nutraceuticals have reasonable claims that can be backed by laboratory and animal testing. Others have claims that exist only in folklore, but many of those claims cannot be substantiated. Evidence does exist that using some of these products in certain doses and at intervals can help the immune response, and many of these compounds would benefit from more clinical investigation.

It is important to look for a reliable manufacturing source. Pills are manufactured in factories, and those factories may not be supervised or certified by the Food and Drug Administration (FDA), the regulatory body in the US. Other countries have their own regulatory bodies. If the manufacturing process is not policed, there is no guarantee that the label, which says the pill contains a certain extract, actually contains it and in the concentrations claimed. If a pill says turmeric, then we need assurance that we are not consuming yellow colored powder. FDA inspections ensure that there is no adulteration. If no one polices the manufacturing process, there is no way to guarantee what the pills actually contain.

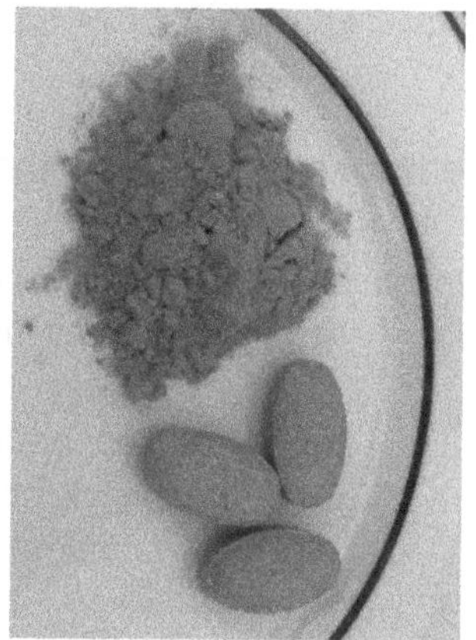

How do you evaluate the claims?

It Is challenging to sift through the claims, so it is worth looking at the source of the information. Does the endorsement come from a non-commercial source or from the person who is selling you the product. The vendor of the supplement might not provide unbiased information since the manufacturer is interested in selling the product. Remember that nutraceuticals are not approved for therapeutic uses by the FDA. They can only be marketed as dietary supplements.

Is it safe to take herbal and other supplements with my cancer treatment?

Resources are available on the websites of major cancer centers such as the Memorial Sloan Kettering Cancer Center in New York, NY, and the Mayo Clinic in Rochester, MN. These provide comprehensive and reliable information about herbal and other supplements.

Resources

- https://www.mskcc.org/cancer-care/treatments/symptom-management/integrative-medicine/herbs
- http://www.mayoclinic.org/drugs-supplements
- Another excellent resource for information is the National Center for Complementary and Integrative Health.
  Their web site is https://nccih.nih.gov.

***

What are alternative therapies?

As opposed to complementary therapy, alternative therapies are used *instead of* conventional therapy. These may consist of:

- Restrictive diets such as the macrobiotic diet.
- Mind-body interventions with Reiki therapy.
- Bio-electromagnetic therapy which is the application of an electromagnetic field using an electric device.
- Nutrition supplements and herbs.

There is no evidence that these work to cure cancer, but patients who choose them over conventional therapy believe that they do. They believe that evidence-based conventional medicine is more invasive and less effective. Unfortunately, studies have shown that patients who choose alternative therapies over conventional therapies have worse survival rates.

One of my patients rejected the recommended chemotherapy for his lymphoma in favor of hydrogen peroxide treatments. He was not forthcoming about where he was getting his information or his treatment. Many doctors tried to reason with him, but he believed that peroxide would cure him. Sadly, it did not, and he succumbed to his cancer. Doctors do agree that chemotherapy is also not always curative, but at least the information about such treatments is transparent. The risks and benefits are established in clinical studies that are published in peer-reviewed journals and are open to discussion.

Other traditional medical systems include Ayurvedic Medicine, Traditional Chinese Medicine, and Naturopathic Medicine. Practitioners of these systems of medicine have received training in schools devoted to that system.

What is Ayurvedic Medicine?

Ayurvedic Medicine is the ancient form of traditional Indian medicine, and it is a medical philosophy that pursues treatment of the whole body not just the disease. This approach may be useful in some chronic illnesses, but it has not been used as a primary treatment in cancer because no clinical trials have established its efficacy. Ayurvedic practices include the use of herbal medicines, mineral or metal supplementation, and the application of special oils using massage. Plant-based treatments in Ayurveda may be derived from roots, leaves, fruits, bark, or seeds such as cardamom and cinnamon. Ayurvedic Medical schools in India exclusively train their graduates in the Ayurvedic tradition, and this form of alternative medicine is widely practiced in India.

What is Traditional Chinese Medicine?

A broad range of medical practices has developed in China based on a tradition of more than 2000 years. They include various forms of herbal medicine, acupuncture, massage, dietary therapy, and exercise. Traditional Chinese medicine is primarily used as a complementary approach in the West. This system emphasizes that disease is caused by disharmony within the functional systems which control digestion, breathing, aging, etc. The herbal preparations used in Chinese medicine may contain an excess of heavy metals which can cause toxic exposure, and regular users need to be aware of this risk.

What is Naturopathy?

Naturopathic practitioners use many different treatment approaches: dietary and lifestyle changes, stress reduction, herbs and other dietary supplements, Homeopathy, manipulative therapies, exercise therapy, practitioner-guided detoxification, psychotherapy, and counseling. Naturopathic practitioners in the United States have attended a Naturopathic School where they receive training in those techniques. Patients often seek out naturopathic treatment for their chronic conditions in addition to routine care from their conventional medicine physician.

What is Homeopathy?

Homeopathy is an alternative medical system developed in Germany more than 200 years ago. It treats diseases using increasingly diluted products, and the mechanism of its action is unknown. There is little evidence of its efficacy in any particular disease, but it continues to be practiced (mainly in Germany and India). Its role in the treatment of cancer has not been established.

***

Some aspects of other traditional systems can be incorporated into complementary therapy. By themselves conventional medicine would consider them to be alternative therapy. There is limited evidence of their success in the treatment of cancer. A few products used in traditional Chinese medicine have shown success in management of some cancers, and they have been studied and developed into successful therapies. Researchers need to pursue promising therapies used in traditional systems and incorporate them into mainstream treatments when they are proven safe and effective.

Anecdotes are not proof...

Many people quote anecdotes about remissions achieved with special teas or other preparations. When we follow diseases with conventional management, there are occasionally apparent remissions in low-grade cancers because the disease waxes and wanes. Some results we cannot explain. We cannot, however, attribute success to interventions that cannot be substantiated by evidence. All treatments should be scientifically studied, and their benefits and toxicity established, before we can recommend or even approve of them.

It is also important to remember that placebo effects can be very powerful. Placebos are compounds or procedures with no known efficacy, yet the user believes strongly that the compound or procedure will work. The human mind is a powerful and still mysterious organ, and scientific evidence shows that it can heal the body in some circumstances. It is quite possible that the anecdotes of remissions represent a successful placebo treatment. Because everyone's mind is different and the placebo compound or procedure may not in itself contribute to the beneficial outcome, we cannot predict that the placebo will help the next patient. This explains why western medicine relies on compounds and procedures proven to be both safe and effective and does not use placebos.

More research is needed...

The National Institutes of Health is studying the benefits and modes of action of complementary and alternative therapies because it is clear that an increasing number of patients are using them. Inform your medical team when you are using such therapies because many complementary therapies can be used with conventional treatments as long as they do not interfere with them.

Neal and Mona looked at their choices. They declined any products that Neal would have to consume that might interact harmfully with his standard treatment. They did seek out massage therapy to help relieve stress, and they said they would consider acupuncture for control of any potential nausea.

Action Plan

- Discuss your complementary therapies with your medical team.
- If you research unconventional medications, consider the source of the information. Discount the information if the source is the vendor selling you the medication.
- Ensure that any complementary therapy does not interfere with the recommended treatment.
- Use alternative therapies with caution.

18. The Mind-Body Connection And a Positive Attitude

What is the connection between your mind and your body?

Is there a connection between how you emotionally react to your illness and the outcome of your treatment? Can you improve your outcome by improving your outlook? According to many holistic medical traditions, the mind-body connection considers the physiological, psychic, and spiritual connections between the state of the body and that of the mind.

Sonia is 85 years old and her blood disorder is being controlled with an oral chemotherapy pill. She visits the doctor for her pre-chemo checkup every month. She is single, and when she comes she is accompanied by her charming twin sister. Sonia continues to teach reading in a local public elementary school. She is always impeccably dressed, always smiling, and never complains of any discomfort.

Gina is 76 years old, and her low-grade chronic leukemia is also being treated with an oral medication. She complains of insomnia and arthritis, is overweight, and has problems related to diabetes. She is always anxious and unhappy in spite of being surrounded by a caring family and a lot of love and support. Each of her clinical visits focuses on urging her to take better care of her overall health, her spirits, and her weight, but Gina continues to spend a lot of time feeling sorry for herself.

These two women cope with their life situations and illnesses very differently. Does Sonia have fewer physical complaints because she has a positive attitude? There may be a connection between their minds and their bodies.

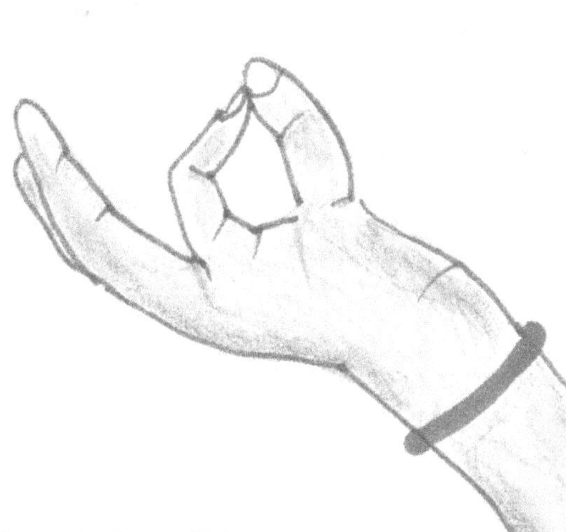

Figure 18.1 Be Mindful

Mindfulness as a way of life can be traced back to ancient Buddhist and Chinese traditions. It teaches people to be aware of their physical and mental being, and it can be a useful tool to cope with physical and mental aspects of cancer and its treatment. Many articles in the popular press have highlighted the benefits of mindfulness and encourage us to be mindful in our daily life whether or not disease is present.

What benefits of mindfulness have been observed in clinical studies?

Weight management: Being mindful of taste and texture of every mouthful of food has helped with weight management. This act of being aware slows down the pace at which you eat your food. Slowing down helps the satiety center in the brain catch up with the amount of food being consumed. Eating quickly without being mindful makes us eat past the point at which we are actually full. Being mindful and feeling satisfied earlier helps limit the amount of food we consume.

Reduction of nausea and anxiety: Being mindful of breathing techniques can help in relaxation, reduction of anxiety, and control of nausea. One such technique is to relax your abdominal muscles and breathe slowly in through your nose until you feel your rib cage expand outwards and your collarbones rise. This fills up the lower part of your lungs. Count slowly to five, and breathe out slowly. Finally push all the air out of your lungs by contracting the abdominal muscles. Repeat several times. This will decrease your heart rate and blood pressure.

Reduction of pain and muscle spasm: Mindful relaxation techniques can help with muscle spasms and pain.

Being mindful and the practice of yoga and meditation have helped manage chronic problems such as hypertension, arthritis, fatigue, and anxiety disorders. Since these practices may help in dealing with some side effects of treatment, they are worth pursuing for that benefit alone.

Does a positive attitude help?

Many people believe that a positive attitude helps fight cancer, but it is unclear whether it actually improves cure rates. A positive attitude does have the important benefit of keeping you engaged in your life. You keep your appointments, follow instructions, and keep up with your exercise and nutrition. You are proactive and get the care that you need. If it were possible for you to keep working, your mind would remain engaged and not be consumed with your cancer diagnosis. All of these actions may help improve survival after a cancer diagnosis.

Published studies have looked at non-cancer causes of death once the patient has received a cancer diagnosis. There was an increase in the incidence of depression, which led to an increase in suicide rates and cardiac deaths. It is very likely that a positive attitude and a good support system would help bring down those rates.

How do you find your balance?

Dealing with a diagnosis of cancer or any other chronic illness starts an internal tug of war for both patients and family members. You may experience anger, sorrow, frustration, and difficulty dealing with this life changing diagnosis. You will need to balance those feelings by the strength needed to endure gathering and processing the information for your illness and proceeding with treatment.

You have to find the balance between being strong for your friends and family and taking help from them.

How do people do it?

- They acknowledge the negatives and focus on the positives.
- They use the resources they have of friends and family, community, and religious affiliations.
- They take advantage of support groups and use meditation and relaxation techniques.
- They keep busy and take time to enjoy small moments and pleasures.
- They call on their inner reserves—even those they didn't know they possessed.
- They decide what is important and what is not.

What is important to you?

A colleague of mine decided to step down from a Director position because it was adding too much stress to her workday and taking time away from her family. Her husband had finally recovered from a major medical procedure.

The anxiety she experienced during his illness clarified her priorities; she wanted to focus only on patient care, not on administrative duties. Being mindful of what was necessary to do her job well and take care of herself and her family helped her make that choice.

Don't sweat the small stuff.

I play recreational tennis with some friends; some fret a lot over line calls and whether the ball is in or out. Because of my daily encounters with grave "end of life" issues, I remind them that we should not get agitated about incorrect line calls (no disrespect intended to professional tennis players). We do our best, acknowledge that some mistakes will be made, and move on. Take this lesson to heart when dealing with a major health issue. Many small things are just not worth upsetting our balance. I have learned this lesson from my patients.

Work is therapy!

Many patients find it therapeutic to keep working and fully engaged and occupied. Work provides a routine and a social structure and keeps your mind off your illness. Unpaid work is just as valuable. Volunteering can also provide a routine, and being useful is very fulfilling.

Work provides an outlet for the caregiver as well. My father suffered from a long and debilitating illness, and my mother was his main caregiver. She set up a complicated system of daily sitters that allowed her to work every day. She changed jobs and moved her home so she could work close by and return on lunch breaks to care for him. She managed to take loving care of him for 10 long years. Work provided a much-needed outlet.

Would a support group help?

Support groups often offer more than emotional support. They can be a valuable resource for practical information. A support group is usually organized by the social worker at the cancer center. You can explore available support groups through the American Cancer Society in the United States or the cancer society in the country where you live. Many support sites are also available online.

Some support groups are organized for different diseases because each cancer site presents its own unique challenges. Families with young children need different kinds of support. People completing their treatments find the transition to being off treatment challenging and need survivorship groups. Patients relapsing from their disease and dealing with prospect of endless treatment are helped by their own cohort.

Not all people need or want to attend a support group. In the beginning, finding the time is itself a challenge. And afterwards some may not want to dwell on the cancer experience and prefer to put it behind them. Others find solace in being able to communicate with others who have faced the same issues. Support groups do not always remain formal either. One of my patient's groups morphed into a knitting circle, and they helped each other through whatever came next.

Some helpful techniques and practices...

Yoga covers a variety of techniques, and its practice has increased around the globe. You can practice it according to your physical capabilities. At a beginner level, simple breathing and stretching exercises can provide health benefits. Look for yoga classes at your local community centers, and many yoga teachers have released instructional DVDs you can follow at home.

Meditation is a self-directed exercise which helps in calming the mind. Many smartphone apps can guide you through the techniques.

Tai Chi and Quigong are Chinese movement, breathing, and relaxation techniques.

Breathwork will help you be aware of your breathing. Full, deep breathing will help you feel relaxed and reduce tension and stress. You can practice breathwork at any time, in any position, and in any place.

Progressive relaxation: When you are in pain, the muscles around the painful area tense up. Learning to relax your muscles can ease the tension in those muscles. One technique is called progressive relaxation. You contract and then relax different muscle groups one by one. For example, start with the foot muscles of one leg. Tense those muscles. Count to ten. Then relax them. Move on to your calf, then your thigh, then your other leg, and so on, up to your belly, back, shoulders, arms, and facial muscles including your jaw. No prescribed order is best.

Guided imagery: The technique called guided imagery encourages you to create a mental picture of a desirable place. Perhaps it is the seashore where you can imagine the feel of the sand between your toes, the spray of the water, the refreshing sea breeze, the warmth of the sun, and the sound of the waves lapping at your feet. You can focus on each sensation and transport yourself to a relaxed state. Your relaxed place can be a green pasture, majestic mountains with snow-capped peaks and crisp mountain air, or it can be your own home, in your comfortable armchair, with a relaxing hot drink and your cozy blanket.

Relaxation for insomnia: When you are worried and have a lot on your mind, you may have difficulty falling asleep and staying asleep. Relaxation techniques can help you fall asleep. If your mind wanders, focus on your breathing. Focus on your body. Relax the muscles and decrease tension they are holding. If you notice certain body parts are tense, you can focus on them to relax them. If your mind wanders again, bring it back to focus on the breathing.

There are many other techniques and interventions. You can pick what suits you best.

Action Plan:

- Stay active and positive.
- Control symptoms with all tools possible: pharmacological and complementary therapies.
- Use your support systems: Family, community, workplace or religious affiliations.
- Enquire about available support groups.

19. Should You Enroll in A Clinical Trial?

Neal and Mona went to the University Center for a second opinion on the treatment recommended by his local cancer team. The specialist at the University Center reviewed his information and agreed that their local oncologist's recommendation was consistent with the current standard of care.

The University specialist then presented another option. They offered Neal the opportunity to enroll in a clinical trial using a different approach. Since this new approach was still in the testing process, no one knew if it was better than the current standard. Neal and Mona had a long discussion regarding the pros and cons of their choices. They were also concerned about the cost of a clinical trial.

What is a clinical trial?

Clinical trials are stepwise approaches to developing new therapies. The first step is to develop new chemical and biologic agents in the laboratory.

Laboratory and Animal Studies: Testing for new drugs to cure cancer takes place first in petri dishes using commercially developed cancer cells. Then the new technique is tried in animals, most of the time in mice. The laboratory or pre–clinical phase can take at least five years and as many as 10 years to complete.

Human Studies: Once scientists have a reasonable expectation of safety and believe they know how the disease will respond, the new drug becomes available for human trials.

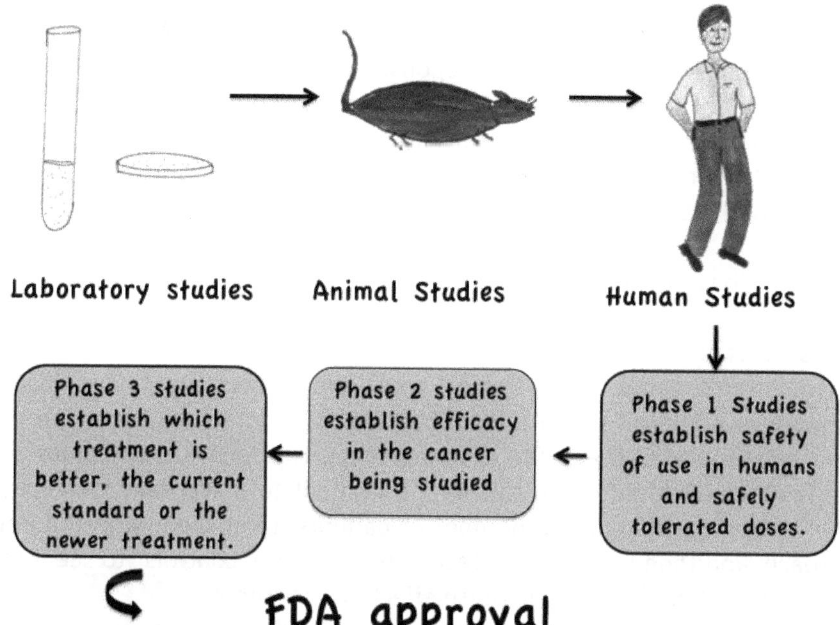

Figure 19.1 Drug Development and Clinical Trials

The Phase 1 Trial:

The Phase 1 trial is the first step in studying how the new drug will react in humans, and that is the only goal at this step. The drugs are given in small doses to the first group of patients. If patients tolerate it, doses are increased in a planned fashion for the next group of patients. This process continues until the dose administered reaches the Maximum Tolerated Dose (MTD).

The goals are: Is the drug safe, what dose is safe, and are there any unexpected reactions in humans?

Phase 1 trials do not evaluate the response of the tumors to the drug. Patients who participate in Phase 1 trials have often gone through multiple standard treatments. When the disease has continued to grow, the patients are willing to take the risk of an untested treatment. Patients should not expect a "miracle cure" because the goal of Phase 1 is to evaluate safety, not efficacy.

It is important to remember that Phase 1 trials are only the first step in using new and innovative compounds in the human body, and they are only attempted after several years of laboratory testing. It is tempting to think of a Phase 1 trial as the possible lottery ticket to a remission, even a cure. According to a study that tracked drug approval rates from 2004-2010, however, the percentage of chemical compounds that will become effective cancer-fighting drugs is one in 20. For biological agents it is one in five. The numbers are better for biological drugs because they target specific proteins, and there have been impressive responses in early trials of some biologic drugs. Chemical compounds act more generally, and their success rate is less.

When you participate in a Phase 1 trial, you move the knowledge base forward. Knowing that your participation will benefit future patients, it may be worthwhile to enroll.

When the Phase 1 "experiment" is successful, the next step is a

» **Phase 2 Trial:**

Based on the results of the Phase 1 trials, the doctors know what dose is tolerated in humans. In Phase 2 trials, the **goal** is to actually measure the disease response to see if the new treatment is effective. Sometimes the trial is designed to compare this new treatment to a standard treatment. Other Phase 2 trials enroll a number of patients, treat them with the new approach, and then compare the results to "historical controls" to see if the new treatment had a better or worse effect on the tumor.

It may be difficult to decide whether you should participate in a Phase 2 trial. Standard treatments may still be available to you, but the odds of their success may be limited. You may want to enroll hoping for a better outcome. Your choices will depend on what trials are available and which ones you qualify for at the time you need treatment.

If the new drug shows reasonable promise of improving current standards of cure when Phase 2 is completed, it moves on to a ...

» **Phase 3 Trial:**

Patients who have the same disease at the same stage are enrolled in Phase 3 trials. A central study board, not the treating physician, assigns either the novel approach or the standard treatment to the patients who are enrolled in the study. There is no guarantee that a patient will receive the new treatment or that that treatment may be better than the traditional treatment. As the Phase 3 trial progresses, the two groups are compared. The **goal** is to test whether the novel approach shows better outcomes. This information then becomes part of the FDA's decision to approve a new drug and of the national organizations' decision to add it to guidelines for treatment. It then becomes the new standard of care.

All current standards of care were developed in this way. For example, in breast cancer, a modified mastectomy proved adequate compared to a radical mastectomy, then a lumpectomy with radiation proved as good as a modified mastectomy, and it became the new standard of care.

Where are the Trials conducted?

All Phase 1 and 2 Trials are conducted in a University or specialty referral center that have active research programs. Phase 3 trials are available in the community setting if the local cancer center participates in such programs.

All trials are supervised and regulated both by the internal cancer committees and tumor registrars and by the external auditors of the trial conducting authority. This insures that no bias favors one or the other treatment. For example, if you gave all your robust patients the stronger treatment, and they had the better outcome, what caused the better outcome? Were the patients in better shape to begin with, or was the treatment better? It is important to have an unbiased answer.

Why do patients enroll?

Some patients enroll because their current and standard treatment has not provided the desired results. The treatment being tested in a trial makes an improved outcome possible. Other patients enroll because they have no other option for standard treatment. They are willing to risk an untested treatment to give them a chance for extending their life.

Who conducts clinical trials?

Several national and international consortia have expert panels that review current treatments and decide what improvements are important and feasible. They design a trial, decide what kind of patients they need to enroll, and determine how many patients are needed to give a valid result. The panel decides in advance how to measure the success or failure of the treatment in question and how to monitor its safety. They decide in advance when to halt a trial if adverse events occur.

The trial design goes through a number of reviews. If it passes, it is offered to the participating hospitals or cancer centers. It must pass through the Institutional Review Board, the IRB, at each facility which decides if it is a reasonable and ethical trial for its institution. The Board carefully reviews consent information. If that passes inspection, only then is the trial "opened" at that institution and offered to patients.

How does a patient enroll?

When making any treatment decision, oncologists evaluate the choice between standard treatment and any available and appropriate clinical trials.

A trial is appropriate if it matches the treatment the patient needs and the treatment the trial is offering. Sometimes a suitable trial has met its enrollment numbers and is closed to new enrollments. Sometimes a trial is only accepting a particular stage of the cancer and that is not what the patient has.

If an appropriate trial is offered, patients are given a packet of information to review and time to review it. Once questions or concerns are satisfied, the patient gives "informed consent." Patients are also assured that they may drop out of the trial at a future date if they decide to do so. There should be no pressure to participate in a trial.

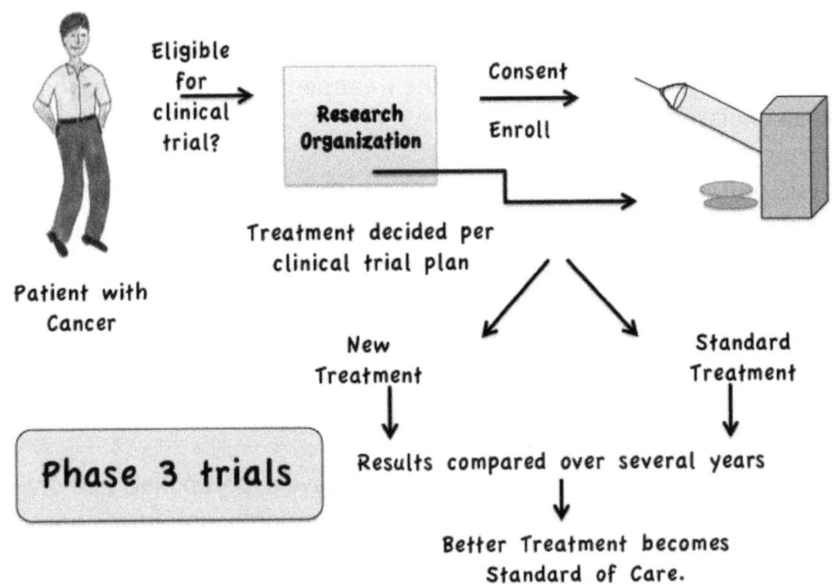

Figure 19.2

The importance of informed consent for trials...

We have come a long way since the days of experimenting on human beings without their knowledge or consent. One egregious example of this is the experimentation done on human beings in the Nazi concentration camps. Another is the Tuskegee Syphilis Experiment where penicillin was withheld from a group of African American men without their knowledge to see how syphilis would evolve if left untreated. A third is the case of Henrietta Lacks, a poor, African-American woman in Baltimore who developed cervical cancer and died from it in 1951. The cells taken from her tumor have been developed commercially into experimental cell lines that have led to many medical discoveries and treatments. Neither Henrietta nor her family knew about this or benefited from the commercialization of her tissue. This would not happen today.

Are experiments on animals necessary?

Several groups would like to do away with experimenting on animals. Unfortunately, one cannot translate the effects of a drug developed in a petri dish to a human being without testing it on animals. In fact, the transgressions of the Nazis and those in the Tuskegee study discussed above led to legislation mandating that no medical treatment be given to humans without first assessing its safety in animals.

The question is what can be done to make sure that animal testing is performed humanely without causing unnecessary pain and suffering. All animal experiments are reviewed and supervised by a committee called the Institutional Animal Care and Use Committee (IACUC).

> All advances in Medical Treatments owe their success both to animal testing and to selfless patients who have enrolled in trials without any personal expectation of gain or guarantee of benefit.

Who pays for the clinical trials?

Clinical trials are expensive. Initially drug development is done in the laboratory and in animal studies. After that human trials need to be conducted for safety and efficacy. This requires millions of dollars to deliver the treatments, to gather the data, and to analyze it over the length of the trial and beyond.

One pathway is provided by research funded by the **National Institutes of Health (NIH) and the National Cancer Institute (NCI).** Academic clinicians submit proposals to study the effects of a drug or an intervention on a specific disease condition. If funded, clinicians recruit patients to the trial of the drug or procedure. Different **National Organizations**, e.g. NSABP (National Surgical Adjuvant Breast and Bowel Program), are dedicated to the study of specific diseases. Their panel of doctors and scientists determines which clinical or treatment question needs to be answered next in order to move knowledge of the disease forward, and they submit grant applications to have it funded. Disease specific advocacy groups also fund specific research, e.g. the Susan G. Komen Breast Cancer Foundation or the Leukemia and Lymphoma Society.

Another pathway is provided by pharmaceutical industry funded research. **Pharmaceutical or Biotech companies** sponsor clinical research involving the drugs that they produce. They seek out clinicians who then recruit patients for these studies. With the decline in NIH-supported funding, pharmaceutical industries are providing a growing percentage of clinical trial funding.

Unfortunately, whether such research can be free of commercial pressure, overt or not, can be open to question. To avoid the taint of bias, trialists are encouraged to post both negative and positive results, not just the results which support the use of the drugs.

In the end, if Neal decides to enroll in a clinical trial, he should have no additional expense.

Should you decide to enroll in a clinical trial?

This decision will depend on what kind of cancer you have, where you are in your disease treatment, what your standard treatment options are, and what kind of clinical trials are available. Will you have to travel for treatment? Is it available locally? What are your resources?

Points to consider:

- Is the disease treatment well standardized by national guidelines, or is it in a state of uncertainty?
- Is a clinical trial available to advance the state of knowledge?
- Will the patient qualify for the trial at the time treatment is needed?
- Can the treatment be delivered locally, or is travel involved?

If you enroll, what is the benefit to you?

The main benefit in enrolling in a trial is contributing to the knowledge base. Your treatment plan is based on previous clinical trials to which other patients contributed by helping to answer the question: Which treatment is more effective? That is a critical piece of cancer research. You may or may not receive treatment that ultimately proves to be more effective. You are enrolling in the trial mainly to further research. It is possible that one of the drugs being tested has the potential to become the next breakthrough.

The luck of the draw...

Sid had developed cancer in his leg bone when he was a teenager. At the time the standard treatment was amputation. Because a treatment was being developed that doctors felt might prevent an amputation, he enrolled in the trial. He was assigned to the amputation group. As the trial progressed, the results showed that the alternate treatment did not work and a number of patients assigned to the alternate treatment died. Amputation remained the standard treatment. This was the value of the clinical trial. Without it, patients and physicians might be tempted to try treatments that did not involve amputation without any proof that those treatments would increase their survival. Survival rates are the measure of any new treatment.

The opposite proved true for the treatment for anal cancer. Here, results of the trials moved the standard treatment away from surgery to radiation plus chemotherapy.

Neal and Mona weighed the options, and they decided to return to their local oncology team and start standard treatment. They kept the option to enroll in a clinical trial for a future date.

Resources:
https://www.clinicaltrials.gov

Action Plan:

- Explore all options with your local Oncologist and with the Oncologist who provides your second opinion.
- Consider a clinical trial if treatment for your condition is not standardized.
- Consider a clinical trial if two treatments are equivalent and they are being compared to see which one is better.

20. How to Handle Fertility Issues?

When patients go through cancer treatment in their childbearing years, they risk becoming infertile and being unable to bear children because of the treatment. The risk of infertility from cancer treatment depends on the type and location of cancer, the type of treatment, the number, type and dose of drugs used, any previous history of infertility, and the age of the patients when they undergo treatment. The effect on fertility may be temporary or permanent.

When to discuss fertility preservation?

So much is happening with a new cancer diagnosis that the preservation of fertility often takes a back seat. With high cure rates and longer life expectancy, however, doctors need to offer this option before cancer treatment begins. Discussing how to preserve the fertility of either sex needs to be part of the treatment planning. The timeliness of the process is easier if a relationship already exists between the cancer center, a fertility specialist, and sperm banks so that quick referrals can be arranged. Cancers that affect people in their childbearing ages are potentially curable, and the possible effect on future childbearing can be important to individuals.

Rita was 27 years old with newly diagnosed Hodgkin's lymphoma. She came for her initial visits with her boyfriend of two years. They were living together and now dealing with her disease together. She had a highly curable cancer, with a good long-term outcome, but she was going to need both chemotherapy and radiation therapy. As we talked about the side effects of the chemotherapy, we discussed the possibility of the treatment making her infertile. In addition to dealing with the lymphoma, the treatment, and their side effects, the couple also needed to think about possible infertility issues and how they might ameliorate them.

After some discussion, Rita decided not to pursue fertility preservation techniques. She completed her treatments, remains disease free, and has resumed her menstrual cycles. She is now engaged to be married to her lovely and supportive boyfriend, now fiancée.

Meera was being treated for fertility issues before her diagnosis of Hodgkin's lymphoma. When she came to see me for treatment of her Lymphoma, neither she nor her husband was interested in additional procedures to preserve fertility given her difficulty in conceiving to begin with. We completed her curative chemotherapy and her normal menstrual cycles returned. To their happy surprise, a few years later she gave birth to two naturally conceived children!

How can one preserve fertility during and after cancer treatments?

Male fertility preservation:

Men have the option of having their sperm collected, frozen, and stored for later use. Sperm banks and the technology used for banking are commonly available. Sperm count and motility will be tested before storage to make sure there are enough live and active sperm available. In pre-pubescent males the possibility of storing testicular tissue for future re-implantation is being explored, but it is not a mainstream technique.

Female fertility preservation:

Women have the option of freezing embryos that is similar to the process for in vitro fertilization (IVF). Eggs are collected, fertilized with a partner's or donor's sperm, and the embryos are frozen for future use. Women now also have the option of freezing oocytes, or eggs, if they do not have a sperm donor. Freezing ovarian tissue, which can be surgically re-implanted later, is being used in select centers. All re-implantation carries some risk of re-implanting cancer cells. This procedure is still considered experimental in pre-pubescent girls.

Collecting enough eggs to create the embryos or to store the eggs used to take at least a month, and oncologists were reluctant to delay the start of curative chemotherapy that long. Now, however, collecting the eggs can be done with a seven-day cycle according to reproductive endocrinologists. This option will not delay cancer treatment too much.

Not everyone becomes infertile after treatment. Normal sperm count and function in males and normal menstrual cycles with ovulation in females can recover. Children conceived after cancer treatment is completed do not appear to suffer harm because of the treatment. When normal sperm production and ovulation resumes, it is not necessary to use the stored sperm and eggs. However, just because your menstrual cycles have started again does not mean that you are ovulating and have regained fertility.

What are the other options?

If Rita's ability to ovulate does not return, what are her other options?

Rita can fertilize the **eggs of a donor** with her husband's sperm and implant those embryos in her own uterus. **Donor embryos** may also be available through fertility centers from couples who have stored extra embryos for their own fertility treatments. If Rita is unable to sustain an implanted embryo, **surrogacy** can be an option. In this process the fertilized embryo is implanted in another woman, and she carries the fetus to term. Laws regulating surrogacy vary by country, so confirm that it is an option where you live. If none of these is available or desired, Rita and her husband can explore the possibility of **adoption.**

Men do have the option of **storing sperm** without the surgical intervention that is required to harvest eggs. If a man's sperm count is low to begin with, sperm storage may not be successful. In that case, **donor sperm** can be used to fertilize their partner's egg. Occasionally sperm can be **harvested directly from the testicles** because the testicles may contain sperm even if it is not present in the semen.

Many of my patients have happily adopted children to complete their families. Others have chosen not to pursue any of the above options.

Resources:
http://www.livestrong.org/we-can-help/fertility-services/

Action Plan

- Discuss fertility preservation options and decide whether they are right for you.
- Ask for a referral to a fertility specialist.
- Consider whether there is adequate time to pursue fertility. treatment before you start cancer therapy.
- Consider your overall life situation.
- Consider counseling.

21. Genetic Testing in Cancer

Does cancer run in your family?

When you come for your first consultation, we ask if there are other members in your family who have had a cancer diagnosis. Often our patients respond, "Cancer runs in my family." In that case we create a family tree noting who got what kind of cancer, at what age, and what the outcome was. Certain patterns can emerge such as early age of diagnosis, multiple cancers within the same person, or the same kind of cancers in a number of close relatives. This information can indicate abnormalities in genes common to family members and inherited from one generation to the next.

Joan is a 39-year-old woman who is in great health. She exercises regularly, maintains a normal weight, has never smoked, eats a healthful diet, drinks alcohol in moderation, and accompanies her 38 year old sister for all her sister's chemotherapy sessions.

Their family tree (See Figure 21.1) is dotted with breast and ovarian cancer diagnoses in multiple generations. Cancer has afflicted her maternal grandmother, that grandmother's sister, Joan's mother, her mother's sister and brother, and now Joan's sister. Joan is considering genetic testing. If she does carry a cancer gene, she wonders what she should do.

Joan meets with the Genetics counselor. After reviewing her family history, they agree that there is a strong risk of an inherited mutation. The counselor asks to test the sister who has had breast cancer to pinpoint the possible genetic mutation. Then she will send Joan's blood for testing. Joan's blood test shows that she is a carrier of the same mutation. She will now evaluate what preventive action she can take so that she does not develop cancer in the future.

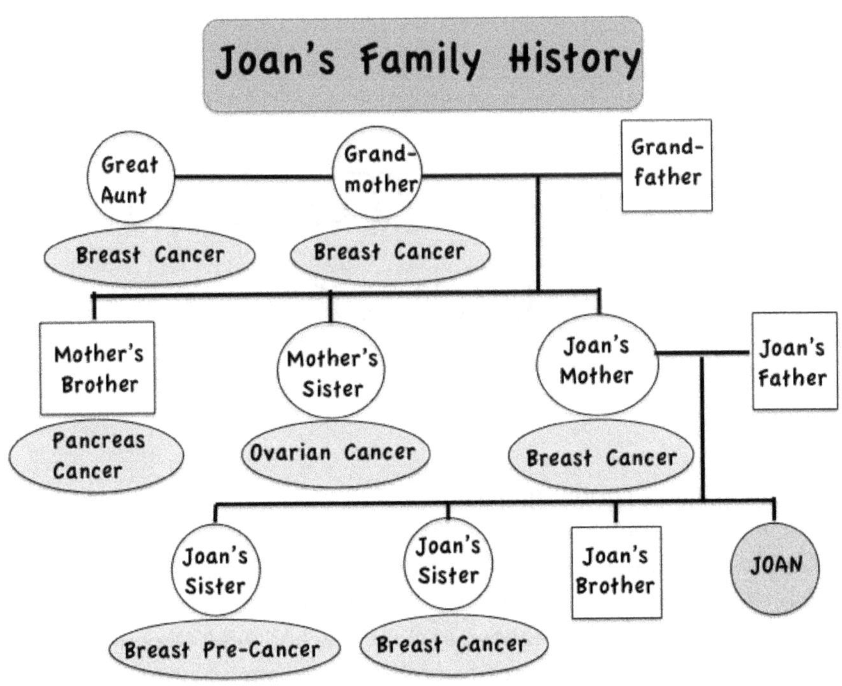

Figure 21.1

What is a gene mutation?

Each person has 23 pairs of chromosomes (22 autosomal pairs of non-sex chromosomes plus one X/Y or X/X pair which determines sex). The chromosomes carry genes which consist of specific sequences of DNA. We carry two copies of each gene--one inherited from each parent on each matched pair. Genes determine form and function of everything from the color of your eyes and shape of your nose to your blood type, metabolism, and immunity. Any of the above characteristics can require one or both of the copies of the gene to function correctly.

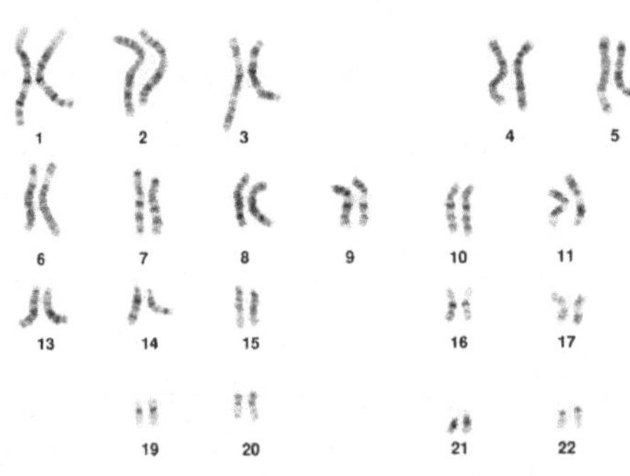

Figure 21.2

A fault or mutation can be present on only one or both copies of a gene. When one faulty copy of the pair is enough to cause a disease, that mutation is called a **dominant** mutation because one bad copy *dominates* the outcome. When both copies must be faulty in order to cause disease, that mutation is called a **recessive** mutation. In this case, the normal gene in the pair can compensate for the faulty gene.

When dominant mutations are inherited, the pathway to cancer is faster and more likely. Since the bad gene is already present, it can trigger cancer at an earlier age than expected. If there is no inherited gene mutation, the defect in the gene has to occur by chance.

Some gene mutations have been clearly linked to the development of specific Cancers. For example:

- **BRCA 1 and 2 mutations** can confer an increased risk of ovarian and/or breast cancer as well as some other cancers. Carrying either one of these mutations can increase the lifetime risk of such cancers in the range of 50 to 90 per cent. These mutations tend to cluster in some ethnic groups, but they do occur in a variety of people. They can be inherited from either the mother's or father's side.
- **Lynch syndrome** causes an increased incidence mainly of colon and uterine cancers. It is caused by a dominant mutation in a gene that repairs DNA.
- **Li-Fraumeni syndrome** causes high rates of early breast cancer, sarcoma, and brain and adrenal gland cancers. It results when one bad copy of a tumor suppressor gene is inherited from a parent.

Why perform genetic testing?

If cancer runs in the family, we wonder how much of that is due to faulty genes or to a faulty environment. Faulty genes or mutations have specifically caused specific family clusters of cancers. For those genetic mutations like the ones described above, family members can take advantage of genetic testing so they can be vigilant. Sometimes they can take preventive action.

The decision to test should be made after a thoughtful discussion regarding the ramifications of such testing. If you know that you carry the mutation and have an almost 100 per cent risk of developing cancer, you may choose to have preventive surgery. This can include removal and reconstruction of breasts, for example, if you test positive for the BRCA mutation. When Hollywood actor Angelina Jolie underwent preventive surgery after she tested positive for the BRCA mutation, it resulted in increased awareness of gene testing. If testing shows that you are at an increased risk of colon cancer, you may start colonoscopy screening at an earlier age. Genetic testing is *only* meant to pick up the specific cancer causing mutation for which you are being tested. It does *not* give you your overall risk for developing any cancer.

Can you lose your insurance or your job if your gene test shows a culprit mutation?

United States law now protects against discrimination if you test positive for a cancer-causing mutation. In 2008 the Genetic Information Non Discrimination Act (GINA) was passed to keep patients from being denied health insurance or employment opportunities because of the results of genetic testing. In addition to cancer, genetic tests may be developed eventually to assess the risk of developing Alzheimer's dementia, diabetes, or heart disease. In addition, when patients participate in clinical studies, genetic testing may uncover mutations that have as yet unknown significance. GINA protects all of us from the results of any genetic testing.

Why does cancer run in my family when we can't identify a genetic cause?

Often, even if cancer runs in your family, researchers have not yet identified the gene mutation that may predispose you to that cancer. That work is ongoing.

Non-genetic reasons can also cause cancer to cluster in families. These may include where we live, the occupations we pursue, the foods we eat, and whether we exercise, smoke, or drink alcohol in excess. We do not have much control over some of these factors. We live and grow up where we do, and we pursue those occupations that are available to us.

We can work at improving our environmental conditions by decreasing pollution and supporting environmental protection. We can improve our personal habits by exercising, not using tobacco, and eating and drinking in moderation. These changes have a direct and measurable impact on our cancer risk independent of genetic mutations.

How do you proceed with genetic testing?

You make the decision to proceed with the genetic test after a discussion with your doctor. You may also have a counseling session with a trained genetics counselor. The result of the test, positive or negative, can have a major impact on your life, and you need to be prepared.

Next, if you want insurance to pay for the testing, you will need to obtain their checklist and get pre-authorization. The genetics counselor will help with that. The tests are expensive and can cost between US $ 2000 and $3000. The test is performed on a sample of body fluid, usually blood, but sometimes saliva. The sample is sent to a specialized laboratory qualified to run these tests. Only a handful of tests are currently available for specific cancers.

What can the results tell you?

The test results can be:

- **Positive**. Yes, you carry the specific gene mutation for which you were tested, and you are at risk for developing that particular cancer.
- **Negative**. No, you do not carry the specific mutation, and your risk for developing that cancer is not increased. Note, however, that the risk is not zero because there are often other unknown risk factors.
- **Variant of Unknown Significance, or Indeterminate**. Some abnormality was detected, but it is unclear whether it will increase the risk of that cancer. This information is entered into a database that is tracked for future incidence of cancer. Eventually it may go into the positive or negative column. At this point we do not know what to do with these results.

The genetics counselor and your doctor will help you sort out the meaning of these results.

Testing your cancer cell for mutations or abnormal genes:

Another kind of genetic testing takes place *after* cancer has been diagnosed. It is not performed for preventive measures. This testing is done *directly on the cancer cell* that was obtained during the biopsy or surgery. Some genetic mutations have been identified that contribute to the growth of the cell. Drugs have been developed to work against those specific mutations. These drugs attack only the intended target. They have minimal impact on the rest of the body's cells so they spare patients the toxicity of chemotherapy. The drugs only work, however, if the cancer cell has the targeted mutation; they would not be effective without it.

This way of treating cancer is gaining ground because more mutations are being identified in the cancer cells themselves that can be targets for drugs designed to work against them. In the coming decades our current treatments using chemotherapy may seem very primitive. They may be replaced by drugs that target genetic mutations of the cancer cell itself.

Fill in your own Family Health Tree.

Neal fills in his family health tree. Some scattered relatives have a variety of cancers, but this does not point to a possible genetic mutation that caused his cancer. They do not need to proceed with genetic testing.

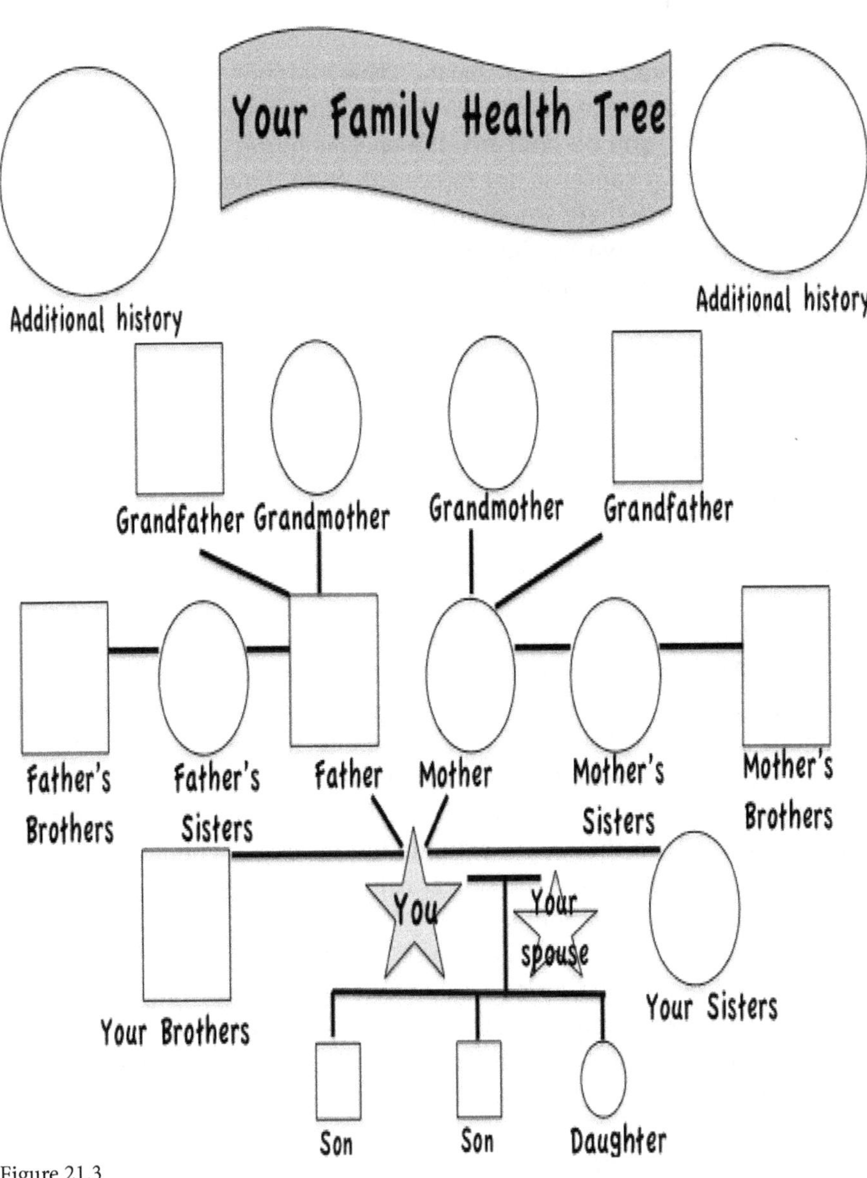
Your Family Health Tree
Additional history
Additional history
Grandfather
Grandmother
Grandmother
Grandfather
Father's Brothers
Father's Sisters
Father
Mother
Mother's Sisters
Mother's Brothers
You
Your spouse
Your Brothers
Your Sisters
Son
Son
Daughter

Figure 21.3

Action Plan:

- Make a family tree of cancer diagnoses.
- Gather information on any family member who was diagnosed and treated for cancer.
- What was their age at diagnosis? What kind of cancer was confirmed and (possibly) at what stage?
- What was the outcome?

Glossary

- Gene= A strand of DNA in specific sequence that carries the genetic code.
- Mutation= A faulty gene.
- Dominant mutation= Only one faulty gene of the pair is required for disease.
- Recessive mutation= Both copies of the pair need to be faulty in order to cause disease.

"Courage is resistance to fear, mastery of fear, not absence of fear."

Mark Twain
Writer

Section E

Beyond The Treatment

22. How Do the Numbers Predict Your Odds?

Why do we use statistics in cancer?

We use statistics constantly in everyday life to measure and predict a variety of things. We consult them to predict the performance of ball players or changes in the housing market. We use our past household expenses to budget for future expenses. In much same way, statistics are used to measure success or failure in cancer. Cancer statistics are a way of keeping score—of calculating the odds both of developing cancer and of beating it.

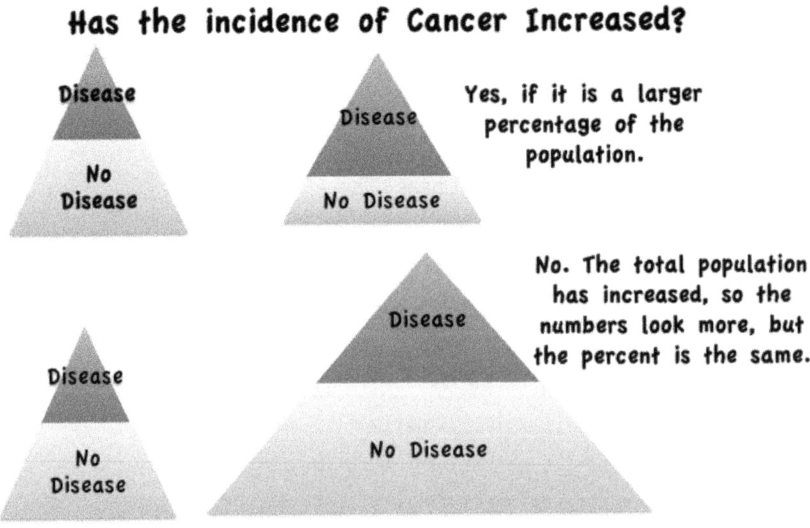

Figure 22.1

How do we use statistics in cancer?

* We measure **Incidence**. As we notice more cancer cases in our friends and family, we often think cancer is becoming an epidemic. It may be, however, that we are seeing greater numbers of cancer patients because the overall population has increased not because the cancer frequency has increased. If we count the number of people developing cancer in any given time period and then convert that figure to a fraction of the total population, if that fraction increases, we know that the actual incidence of cancer (and risk) is increasing. If the fraction is not growing, then the cancer risk is not growing even if the number of cases we see around us appears to be increasing. (See Figure 21.1).

* We measure **success** of the treatment in different ways: Five-year survival, overall survival and response rates.

What is five-year survival?

In cancer literature doctors talk about different kinds of survival. The most common benchmark is the **five-year survival rate** when doctors believe the patient has been *cured* because he/she has lived disease free for five years. When additional (or adjuvant) treatment is added to the initial curative treatment, the need for such treatment is justified by an improvement in five-year survival rates. Both aggressive cancers and most low-grade cancers will relapse within that period of time if they are going to do so. If the patient's cancer has not recurred after five years, doctors consider it reasonable to assume that it would not relapse in the future. It has became a predictor of long-term cure.

Another measure of success of the treatment is an improvement in **overall survival** rates. In Stage 4 cancer cure rates cannot be measured. A patient may survive only two years, but two years might be longer than most patients survive that kind of cancer, and the treatment may represent success.

A third measurement that oncologists use concerns the percentage of tumors that respond by shrinking (**response rates**).

In some kinds of cancer, once you are disease free for two-years, the odds get dramatically better. In some others, you must be disease free for seven to ten years. The length of time for others extends to 20 years.

How do we know that new treatments are better?

Researchers and doctors measure the success rates of the treatments being compared. Depending on the type of cancer, the stage, and the treatment being considered for it, the measure of success may be five-year survival, disease free survival, overall survival, or response rates of the tumor.

For example, in a clinical trial comparing two treatments X and Y, a certain number of patients are given treatment X and a similar group of patients is given treatment Y. The results are compared. If treatment X was better than treatment Y, X gets the nod of approval.

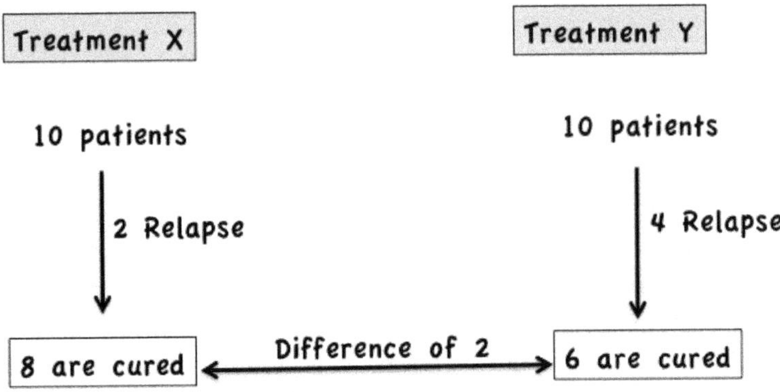

Is Treatment X really better than Treatment Y?
Are the patients in the Y group sicker and therefore do worse?
Is it chance?

Statistical analysis is needed for the answer.

Figure 22.2

Statistics tell researchers how many patients to enroll in a study in order to say that the difference achieved was because of a better treatment and not because of chance alone. If only 10 patients were enrolled in each group, and eight of 10 patients in group X had a good outcome compared to six of 10 in group Y, can the improvement of only two patients be attributed to treatment X, or can it be caused by other variables? Were those two patients healthier? Younger? Did their disease grow more slowly? This is where statistics (or biostatistics, in this sort of statistics) is important. It tells us beforehand how many patients we need to enroll and how big the difference needs to be in order for the results to be meaningful. Without this, we do not have a winner. This sort of analysis is important in all branches of medicine, but it is critical in the treatment of cancer.

When can you say you are cancer free?

After **curative** treatment patients wonder, "At what point am I cancer free? Do I have to wait five years to know?" Unfortunately, there is no uniform answer to that question. I like to think my patients are cancer free after they finish their initial treatment. In my opinion, when there is no disease to measure, we should consider it gone.

***

Recently a patient who had Stage 4 cancer came for his pre-chemotherapy checkup. When he was first diagnosed, he had asked me how long he had to live. While we do not know what actual length of time an individual will survive, the statistics give us an estimate. My patient was told that he had approximately a year. After fourteen months he was doing well, but he was waiting for his time to be up. Well, that is not how it works. There is no clock that starts the countdown. If you are doing well, you can continue to do well. The statistics are not a crystal ball.

***

Sports statistics tell us about what we might expect from a particular player judging from his/her past performances, but they do not guarantee that the performance will be repeated. Statistics are valuable because they give us a general prediction, a way of comparing treatments, and the ability to give patients some idea of where they stand.

Cancer statistics also give both doctors and patients a general prediction of success according to the type, stage, and other characteristics of the cancer. There is always variability in outcomes, but the general prediction is a good place to start.

Action Plan

- Know your odds because they will guide your decision.
- Remember the odds are only a guide, not a certainty.

23. Beyond Cancer... Survivorship.

You have finished your treatment. What happens next?

The last few months have been intense. You have faced your mortality and succeeded in overcoming innumerable challenges. You are now on the road to recovery, getting back to your previous routines, and perhaps instituting some new ones. Life will get back to normal or you will find a new aspect of normal life. You are celebrating, but the joy is tinged with anxiety. You have been extremely busy with treatments and appointments and side effects and medication lists. You have been supported by your team--the doctors and nurses, the phlebotomist, the radiation therapist--and you have felt taken care of. Now the daily appointments and phone calls have ceased, and you can return to your family, your work, and other aspects of daily life.

This is a period of transition and anxiety. Who will be watching you closely? How will you know if the cancer returns? You need reassurance. Even though your treatment has been completed, and you won't be talking to your team constantly, they are still available for questions.

Follow up visits

You will continue to have routine appointments with your oncologists. Depending on your kind of cancer, you will be scheduled for scans and blood work on a prescribed schedule. In combination with your checkups, the scans and blood work will monitor you for any relapse. You can always call your doctor if you notice that something is different. Your team will keep up this surveillance for at least the next five years--sometimes longer.

Survivorship Care Plan

At the end of your active treatment, you should get a written summary of the treatments that you received. It should contain the names and dates of your treatments, any dosage adjustments, and any major side effects from which you suffered. It should also contain the plan of care for follow up and surveillance. This is your blueprint about what to expect and what to watch for. It is particularly important if you move to a different city or state because you can carry this information to your new doctors. If you do move, also carry the images of your scans on a disc, not just the reports. Your new facility will need them for comparison.

Consult the example of the Survivorship Care Plan developed by the American Society of Clinical Oncology provided in the Appendix. Your center may use several of such templates.

What is Survivorship?

Unlike the commonly used term and badge of honor of "surviving" your cancer, survivorship concerns dealing with the aftermath of the cure. We have started diagnosing, treating, and, thankfully, curing many cancers in younger patients. In the treatment's aftermath, patients now have a long lifespan, and they may need to deal with the long-term side effects of their treatment.

The Survivorship Clinic provides a combination of services for a variety of issues:

- **Psychological help** to address the anxiety and depression caused by dealing with the possibility of a recurrence of your cancer. It is not unusual to experience emotional distress similar to PTSD (Post Traumatic Stress Syndrome) or separation anxiety from your team. You may be anxious about the results of your surveillance. For some people, completion of the surveillance protocol and being discharged from oncology care is distressing. I have patients who are delighted to be discharged and patients who prefer to keep coming for an annual visit even if they are disease free.
- **Fertility issues** when sterility is caused by surgery, radiation, or medicines.
- **Sexual dysfunction** that occurs for multiple reasons.
- **Nutrition problems** that result from difficulty swallowing, loss of salivary function, or surgery on the stomach or intestines.
- **Cardiac** follow-up for coronary disease resulting from chest radiation or chemotherapy drugs.
- **Breathing difficulty** from lung scarring.
- **Other medical Issues**: Strokes or blood clots, anemia, kidney malfunction, or lymphedema.
- **Loss of functioning** that leads to unemployment and financial problems.

Many people move on. They are happy to be cured. Life has changed, but they deal with it. Others need more help. If we recognize the problems, then we can help with some of them.

Resources:

- If your cancer center does not have a survivorship service, a number of resources are available online.
- The Livestrong Care plan: http://www.livestrongcareplan.org/

A sample Survivorship Care Plan is provided in Appendix 4.

Cancer Prevention

As a survivor, what can you do to decrease your risk of recurrence? In addition to improving your own outcome, these measures will also help your family members decrease their risk of developing cancer.

- **Avoid Tobacco Use**

Tobacco in all its forms has been associated with cancer. Chewing tobacco or snuff tobacco increases the risk for cancers of the head and neck. Smoking increases the risk for lung and esophageal/stomach cancer. Patients are surprised to learn that smoking is also associated with bladder cancer. The by-products of tobacco smoke enter our circulatory system and are excreted in the urine. Since the urine stays in the bladder for several hours at a time, the tobacco by-products damage the cells in the bladder lining which can contribute to cancer.

Tobacco use causes many other non-cancer related diseases which can greatly decrease your ability to function including diseases of the heart and circulation, high blood pressure, and strokes. Once children pick up the habit, it is a tough one to kick. We must make it impossibly difficult for children to start both by preventing their access to tobacco and providing education. It is still beneficial for smokers who develop cancer to give it up. The risk for oral, esophagus, and bladder cancer is cut in half five years after quitting, and the risk of lung cancer is cut in half in 10 years.

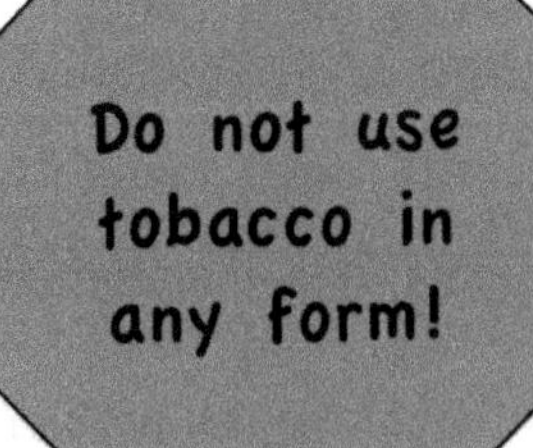

Figure 23.1

As you go through cancer treatment, encourage your family members to quit smoking. I am always astonished at how many of my patient's children continue to smoke even as they bring their parents for radiation and chemotherapy.

Quit Smoking Programs exist in every hospital, and your cancer center will have information on local resources.

- **Limit Your Alcohol Use**

The US Federal Government's *Dietary Guidelines for Americans 2010* define moderate alcohol drinking as up to one drink per day for women and up to two drinks per day for men. They define heavy drinking as having more than three drinks on any day or more than seven drinks per week for women, and more than four drinks on any day or more than 14 drinks per week for men.

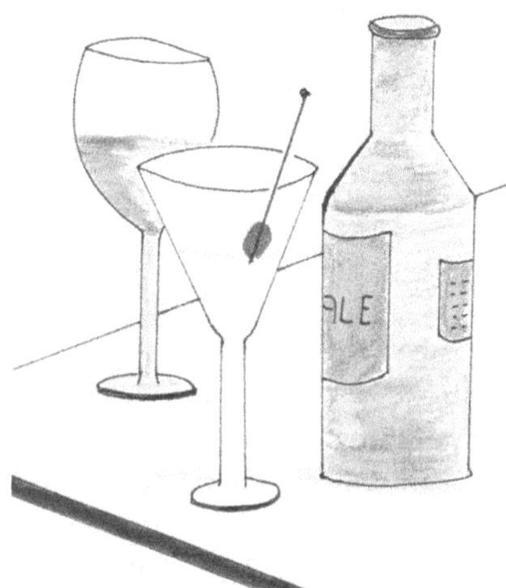

Figure 23.2 .

Alcohol is a major risk factor for cancers of the head and neck, esophagus, and liver. Using tobacco with alcohol multiplies this risk. Regular alcohol consumption also increases the risk of breast cancer and colon cancer. Alcohol's by-product, acetaldehyde, is a toxic chemical, and alcohol impairs the body's ability to absorb a variety of beneficial nutrients. The process of fermentation can also cause accumulation of cancer-causing contaminants. The goal of cancer prevention would be to limit the consumption of alcohol to moderate levels.

- **Take a Baby (81 mg) Aspirin Daily**

Using aspirin has been an attractive avenue of cancer prevention because It is inexpensive and mostly safe. Aspirin is used routinely and effectively to reduce deaths from cardiac disease and strokes. Several recent studies have strengthened the observation that a daily, low-dose aspirin reduces the risk of dying from cancer by almost one third when taken for long periods of time. The real benefit accrues beyond the 10-year mark. The benefit has been associated with daily use, not intermittent use or even taking it every other day, and taking aspirin has to be balanced against the potential risk of gastritis (stomach irritation) and bleeding.

The studies include observational as well as interventional studies. Patients taking a daily aspirin for stroke and heart attack prevention were followed, and those patients who then developed cancer were identified. Compared to patients who took a placebo, aspirin reduced the spread of cancer by a third.

At this time we would recommend a baby aspirin (81 mg) for the long term. If you have a history of bleeding problems, blood count abnormalities that would put you at risk for bleeding, or if you are using other blood thinners, check with your primary doctor to make sure that you can add aspirin.

- **Limit Sun Exposure**

Sun exposure and sunburn increases your risk for skin cancer. Protect yourself from UV rays on both sunny and cloudy days. Limit your exposure by wearing sunscreen with a minimum SPF of 15, avoid tanning beds, limit sun exposure between 10 am and four pm, stay in the shade, and cover up by wearing long sleeved shirts and long pants, a wide brimmed hat, and sunglasses. People who live in hot, sunny climates have developed a culture of covering up and staying indoors during the hot afternoon hours. This is especially important for children because sun exposure at a young age has been linked to skin cancer in adults.

Use:

* Sun Screen lotion.
* Hats.
* Sunglasses.
* Limit sun exposure between 10 am and 4pm.

- **Increase Consumption of Fruits and Vegetables**

Vegetables and fruits protect against a range of cancers including mouth, pharynx, larynx, esophagus, stomach, lung, pancreas, and prostate. They contain vitamins and minerals that help keep the body healthy and strengthen its immune system. They are also good sources of substances like phytochemicals that can help to protect cells from damage that can lead to cancer.

Increased fiber intake also reduces the risk of cancer. Whole-grain bread and pasta, oats, vegetables, and fruits speed up the length of time it takes food

Sunscreen
Protect yourself from the Sun's UV rays

Figure 23.3

Eat the rainbow!

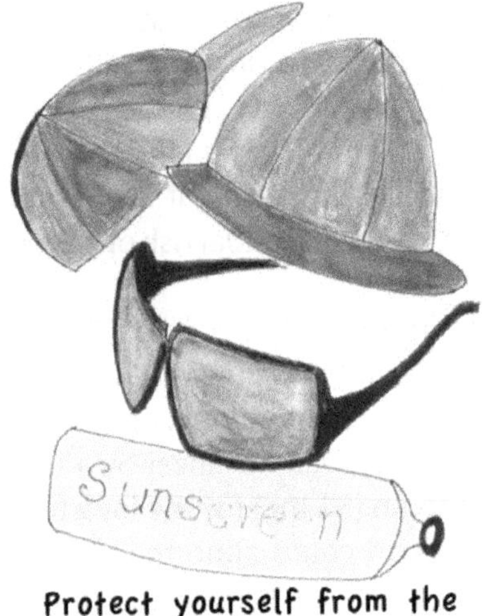

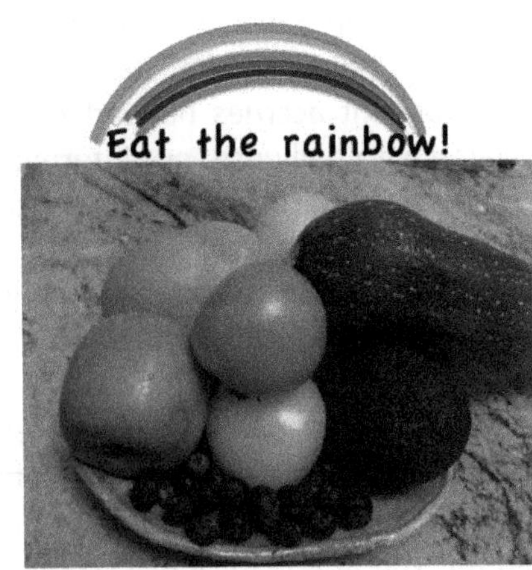

Figure 23.4

to move through the digestive system. This decreases exposure to potential cancer-causing substances in our diets.

We should aim to fill two-thirds of our plate with fruits, vegetables, beans, and whole grains.

Should you take vitamin supplements?

It is better to consume adequately nourishing food and drink which contain the recommended daily allowance of necessary vitamins than to take vitamins. Excess doses of some vitamins have even contributed to increased cancer risk. Real whole foods contain fiber, vitamins, minerals, and phytochemicals. It is better to fill your plate with a variety of vegetables, fruits, whole grains and beans, and one-third (or less) of animal protein.

Sometimes it is necessary to take supplements when you are pregnant or are frail, elderly, or have digestive issues that limit your consumption of a full and balanced diet. Some conditions interfere with absorption of nutrients, and these need to be treated with vitamins. Please note these instructions are for those who are not on active anti-cancer treatment.

- **Increase Physical Activity**

Physical activity in any form helps to lower cancer risk. Aim to build more activity, like brisk walking, into your daily routine. One of my patients gets off a few subway stops earlier than she needs to and walks the rest of the way. Another patient and her co-workers purchased a treadmill and installed it in their lunchroom. Since they had easy access to an exercise machine, they could work exercise into their break times. I always walk places when I can, take the stairs, and park as far away as I can in parking lots. I try to get my exercise early in the morning before work; otherwise too many other tasks get in the way. On days I am slow to move (we all have those days), I give myself permission to exercise only 10 or 15 minutes. Once I start, I can usually keep going. If you are just starting to exercise, build up slowly. Shorter bouts of activity are just as beneficial; it's the total time that counts.

Some people find it motivating to track their physical activity with wearable devices. You can program these devices to remind you to get up and move. Sharing your information with designated friends can provide friendly competition and increase your activity levels.

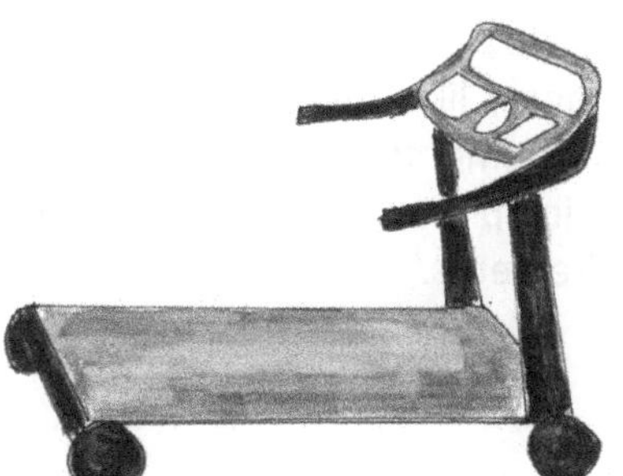

Figure 23.6

- **Limit Your Sedentary Habits.**

One of my patient's tricks to keep active while watching her favorite TV shows is to get up and do jumping jacks during commercial breaks. People's jobs now involve sitting in front of a computer all day long. Such prolonged times of sitting contribute to obesity, and getting up and moving helps with weight control. My husband uses a device that raises and lowers his computer at his desk. Several times a day he will convert the desk to the standing position.

- **Maintain a Healthy Body Weight:**

Body Mass Index (BMI) is one common method used to measure obesity. BMI is a measure of body fat based on a person's weight and height. The BMI chart shows four ranges: underweight, healthy, overweight, and obese. Staying within the healthy range throughout life is important for lowering cancer risk. Another simple way to predict risk is to measure your waist immediately above your hip bone. **For women a waist measurement of 31.5 inches or more indicates high risk. For men a waist measurement of 37 inches or more indicates high risk.** The waist circumference is important because doctors have proved that carrying excess fat around our waists can be particularly harmful. It is strongly linked to colon cancer and to post menopausal breast cancer.

How much activity is good?

The target should be about 30 minutes of vigorous activity or 60 minutes of moderate activity daily. These recommendations change with new findings, but that is a good starting point.

A number of my patients work in jobs involving manual labor like landscaping or construction, and they do not need to invest extra hours in physical exercise. What they need to guard against is relaxing in the evening with a six-pack of beer while watching TV. Jumping Jacks are not required.

Does yoga constitute exercise?

I asked this question of a noted yoga researcher. He said, "If the kind of yoga you are practicing is a half hour of vigorous poses like sun salutations which raise your heart rate for a sustained period of time, this would satisfy your exercise requirement. Other forms of yoga, in spite of all the other health benefits, would not fulfill your exercise requirements."

Can vaccines prevent cancer?

Some viruses are established causes of, or have strong associations with, some cancers. Using the vaccines that have been developed to prevent the viral infection and the associated chronic organ damage will cut down on the incidence of the corresponding cancers.

Chronic Hepatitis B virus infection can lead to primary liver cancer (hepatocellular carcinoma). Since limited treatment is available for liver cancer, prevention of Hepatitis B infection goes a long way in cancer prevention.

The Human Papilloma Virus or HPV is an established cause of cervical cancer. HPV is a common virus and easily transmitted with minor sexual contact. Once HPV enters the tissue and infects the DNA, it is never eliminated, so prevention of the primary infection would cut down on the incidence of cervical cancer. Vaccination is recommended for both girls and boys, and the ideal time to administer the vaccine is before they become sexually active. Unfortunately that age is earlier than parents will want to admit, but the reality is that sexual activity is reaching younger age groups and increasing the risk of HPV transmission. Parents of boys may be complacent because boys will not get cervical cancer. But HPV is implicated in other cancers that affect more men than women like cancers of the throat and anus. Vaccinating boys and girls would protect everyone and decrease rates of HPV transmission.

Throat or head and neck cancers were classically associated with smoking and drinking. In the last ten years, however, a new population (mostly men) has been diagnosed with these cancers, even those men who never smoked or drank alcohol. HPV has been implicated. The treatment for head and neck cancers, a combination of radiation and chemotherapy, is truly one of the most difficult to get through. It is debilitating and has long-term consequences. Throat cancer is sometimes treated with surgery that is radical and requires skillful reconstruction.

Other viruses are associated with some lymphomas or oral cancers, e.g. the Epstein Barr Virus or EBV. No vaccines prevent the EBV infection yet. When they are developed, they will be a boon to cancer prevention.

Action Plan

- Limit alcohol, red meat and processed meat.
- Increase vegetable, fruit and whole grain consumption.
- Avoid tobacco.
- Stay active. Exercise 30-60 total minutes daily.
- Consider a baby aspirin daily.
- Consider available vaccinations.
- Limit sun exposure.

24. When You Decide You Do Not Want Treatment...

When you defined the Goals of Your Treatment in Chapter 14, we mentioned briefly that some patients would not benefit from anti-cancer treatments. If you learn that you are one such patient, and you choose not to pursue any treatment, what are your other options? You may be offered palliative therapy or hospice care, and we will discuss those options in this chapter.

My friend *Reena* called me in some distress; she didn't know what to do. Her 90-year-old father had just been diagnosed with metastatic cancer. He had been very active and self-sufficient until recently when he began to have pain in his hip and difficulty walking. A hip X ray showed that cancer had invaded his bone, and a biopsy confirmed the diagnosis. Doctors evaluated his current condition, his age, the stage of his disease, and his life expectancy. They determined that any cancer treatment would not be curative and might not even extend his life. It would certainly cause side effects and decrease his quality of life. Reena's father had decided against pursuing any treatment, but she was worried about his pain management. She wanted to make sure he would be comfortable and would not suffer. Her father wanted to stay in his home, in familiar and comfortable surroundings, and Reena needed help to make that happen. We discussed the options his doctors had offered him.

Reena's father accepted a short course of radiation treatment to help his painful hip. He decided against chemotherapy because of his age and the stage of his cancer, and he chose to start hospice services.

What is the difference between palliative care and hospice care?

Palliative care treats the symptoms that both the disease and its treatment cause, and doctors offer it at any time during the course of your illness. The presence of a tumor can cause pain or swelling, loss of appetite and weight, nausea, diarrhea or constipation, and a variety of other symptoms that need to be actively managed. Palliative care can also include mild chemotherapy or a short course of radiation therapy whose goal is to manage a specific symptom.

Hospice care is offered to a patient who is near the end of life, and its purpose is to make that journey easier for you and your family. When you are on hospice, the expectation is that you do not want doctors and nurses to use heroic measures in response to a medical emergency. Resuscitating your heart or lungs or placing you on life support at this point would not be helpful in improving your quality of life. Patients with end stage cancer would not be expected to recover from the failure of their vital organs. If they are placed on life support machines, they might spend the rest of their time on those machines.

At the initial consultation with the hospice service, you and your family will learn about the goals of hospice care. You will sign advance directives that you keep at home and at the hospital stating that you do not wish specified life support measures. Instead of calling 911 and going to the emergency room, you will be asked to call the hospice nurse who will come to your home. He/she will assess your situation and consult with your doctors by phone. They will make the necessary adjustments to your medications or adjust plans for your care and comfort. If you have a temporary and treatable condition like a urinary tract infection or bronchitis, you will be treated for it. If you cannot be kept comfortable at home, they will arrange for you to be admitted to a facility specializing in hospice care.

Nurses from the Visiting Nurses Association (VNA) check on me at home. Do I need hospice nurses as well?

The missions of VNA and hospice are different. Visiting nurses are helping to treat a condition that is expected to improve or at least remain stable. If you go home after an operation and need your wound checked, for example, nurses from the VNA will visit until your wound heals. If your high blood pressure is not controlled, the VNA can come to your home and monitor that. They provide services that help you get stronger and better such as delivering physical therapy. If your condition gets worse, they will ask you to go to the hospital for further care because they cannot provide additional services including the type of medicines that will keep you pain free and comfortable towards the end of your life.

If you have a condition like Stage 4 cancer, and you are not expected to get better with any more treatment, hospice services are better at giving you the type of care you need than the VNA. The hospice mission is to take care of you as the disease progresses. Conditions other than cancer, like advanced heart disease, liver failure, or kidney failure, also qualify for hospice services. Hospice services are for all patients whose conditions are expected to worsen and will eventually cause their death. They are not only for the elderly.

Sometimes VNA and hospice services are different arms of the same agency, and the nurse from the VNA can transition with you to hospice. The VNA may have a "bridge to hospice" program where you can begin to receive some benefits of the hospice program until you are ready for full Hospice services.

Who will be my doctor?

Many patients and their families fear that if they decide against active anti-cancer treatment, they will navigate the rest of the journey by themselves. That is not the case. Your doctors will help you whatever your choice may be.

If you have an active relationship with your oncologist, she may remain your physician and coordinate your care with the Hospice agency that will help you at home. If you have a stronger relationship with your Primary doctor, your Primary doctor may take on that role. The hospice agency will also have a Medical Director who will oversee all the care they provide.

Will I be able to stay at home? What kind of services does hospice provide?

If you have signed on with hospice, the hospice nurses and support services will visit you at home. They will assess your needs and your resources, report back to your doctor, and together they will help meet your needs.
Hospice and your doctor will:

- Help with pain management. They will provide what works best for you be it liquid medications, pills, patches, or pumps for continuous infusions. They can increase or decrease the medication as needed.
- Arrange for whatever supportive equipment you may need: a hospital bed, a bedside commode, or oxygen, among other things.
- Arrange for a home health aide to visit if you need some help bathing or with other personal care.
- Help to fill your prescriptions and arrange with their designated pharmacy for home delivery.
- Provide emotional support from volunteers, chaplains, and social workers.

The hospice team will help your family care for you. Their goal is to keep you comfortable and pain free in your chosen environment and to avoid medical intervention that will not benefit you. Hospice will be your point of first contact. They will guide you through the expected changes in your condition.

I live alone. How will I manage?

Hospice will help assess your needs and your resources. If friends, family, neighbors, or others can help with some of your needs, hospice will do its best to fill in the gaps. Hospice does not provide 24-hour home care. If you do need such care, hospice will help arrange admission to a nursing home or hospital facility that can provide hospice level care, and hospice will continue to supervise your care while you are there. If you wish to continue to stay at home and need 24 hour nursing care, you do have the option of hiring nurses from a home care agency in addition to receiving Hospice care.

Can I still see my doctor?

Whether or not you can still see your doctor depends on your agency, and you should discuss that at your initial consultation. It also depends on the condition for which you are on hospice. If you are on hospice for terminal cancer, but you need to visit your Cardiologist for heart failure caused by your cardiac condition, you may be able to do so. You should discuss this kind of issue with your hospice nurse first because she may be able to save you a visit by taking care of it at home. Your doctor is always informed of any change in your condition and has input into your plan of care.

How will I pay for Hospice?

In the United States, Medicare, Medicaid, and most insurance programs cover Hospice services through approved agencies, and you will not have to pay additional fees. Hospice services through government and private programs are available in other countries. The payment system varies by country.

When should I sign on with Hospice?

In general, people qualify for hospice when they have a life expectancy of less than six months, but it will depend on your own situation. Doctors can give an approximate range of time for survival, but it is obviously a rough estimate and can change either with or without treatment. As we spoke about in Chapter 14 on the Goals of Treatment, you and your medical team should have this conversation when treating metastatic disease.

In the past when you signed on with hospice, you also needed to decide that you would not have any cancer treatment. You received treatment for care and comfort only. Regulations have been modified to allow some cancer treatment for symptom relief. Discuss this possibility at your initial consultation with hospice.

Some patients with Stage 4 disease may choose to start Hospice services at the beginning of their disease diagnosis. Depending on a patient's life expectancy, how he is expected to respond to treatment, and his goals for his remaining time, some may choose not to pursue any active cancer treatment. Others may choose to try some treatment and start hospice only if their disease progresses and their condition worsens. The conversation about life expectancy and goals of treatment should not be left until the end. Studies show that patients in hospice experienced a better quality of life at the end.

Resources:

- The National Hospice and Palliative Care Organization. http://www.nhpco.org/about/hospice-care
- The National Hospice Foundation. http://www.nationalhospicefoundation.org

Action Plan:

- Discuss life expectancy and goals of treatment.
- Consult with Hospice.
- Complete Advance Directives and Health Care Proxy.

“Calm mind brings inner strength and self-confidence, so that’s very important for good health.”

Dalai Lama

Section F

Epilogue

Epilogue

We have followed Neal through his initial hospitalization, diagnosis, investigations, and consultations. He sought a second opinion, considered a clinical trial, evaluated his life situation and his goals of treatment, and finally he started the recommended treatment. Scans will assess his response to that treatment. Neal will then be scheduled for ongoing checkups and continue with surveillance. Further treatment decisions will be made according to the results of that surveillance.

Everyone's cancer journey is unique. Every cancer is different, and each patient's response to treatment varies. You may have begun to read this book immediately after your diagnosis or at a variety of other points along your journey. You may be reading it to inform yourself or to help a friend or family member make decisions. I hope the information I have shared either has helped you or will help you make informed choices about difficult decisions and make your journey easier.

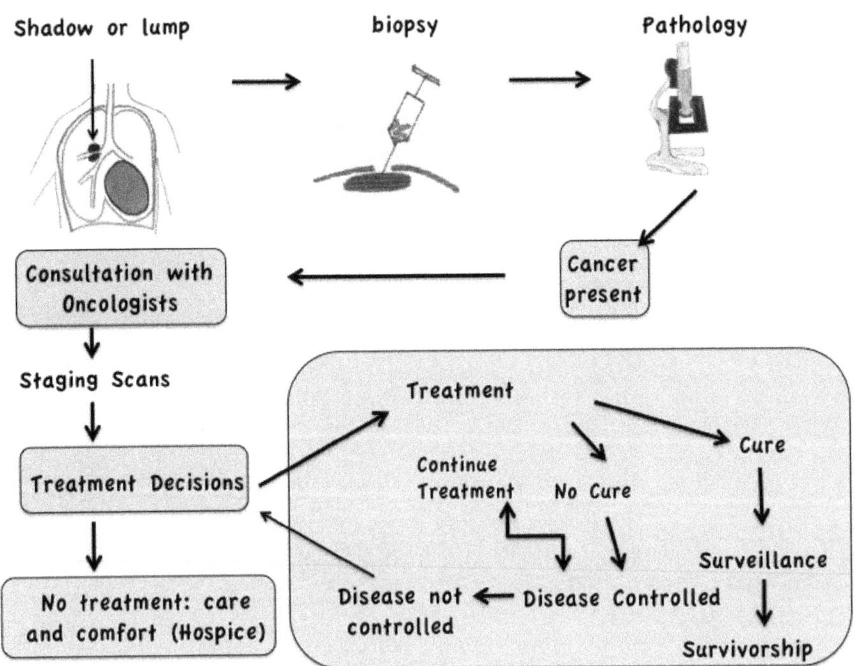

Figure 1. A Patient's Journey

Section G

Appendices

"I love those who can smile in trouble, who can gather strength from distress, and grow brave by reflection."

Leonardo da Vinci
Artist, Scientist, Inventor

APPENDIX 1

1. *Keeping Your Records: Checklists.*

As you start collecting the information you will need for your medical team, these checklists will help you keep track of that information. They cover the diagnosis, consultations, scans and procedures, treaments, medications, and doctor and pharmacy information.

Tasks	✓	**Notes**
Type of Cancer		
Stage of Cancer		
Consultations:		
Radiation Oncology		
Surgical Oncology		
Medical Oncology		
Second Opinion		
Nutrition		
Genetics Counselling		
Financial Counselling		
Treatment Planning		
Clinical Trials ?		
Teaching Session		
Dental Care		

Tasks	✓	Notes
Immunization		
Transportation		
Supportive Care		
Social Worker		
Physical Therapy		
Support Group		
Acupuncture		
Massage Therapy		
Reiki Therapy		
Personal Planning		
Medical Leave		
Human Resources/ Disablility Insurance		
Wills		
Health Care Proxy		
Advance Directives		

Physican Information

Name of MD	Office Address	Office Phone/ Fax	Office Hours

Procedures

Name Of Procedure/ Operation	Date of Procedure	Post Procedure Instructions	Result	Doctor/ Contact

Scans

Name of Scan	Date of Scan	Result	Date of Next Scan
Ultrasound			
Mammogram			
CT Scan Chest			
CT Scan Abdomen			
CT Scan Pelvis			
CT Scan/ MRI Brain			
MRI			
PET Scan			
Bone Scan			

Treatment: Chemotherapy

Date	Blood Test Result	Chemotherapy Drugs	Post Chemo Drugs/Injections

Treatment: Radiation

Dates of Treatment	Area Radiated	If With Chemo-Name of Drugs	Interruptions/ Complications	Total Dose

Additional Notes:

Pharmacies

Name of Pharmacy	Address	Phone/ Fax
Local		
Mail Order		

Medications:

Name of Medicine: Brand/ Generic	For what Symptom?	How to take?	Refills (Y/N); When to renew

Hospitalizations

Name/Address of Hospital	Dates	For what Reason?	Outcome

APPENDIX 2

2. Common Medicines You Will be Prescribed.

You will receive a number of prescriptions to control your symptoms. Often the medications are referred to by their brand names but are filled at the pharmacy as generics. When you need to take the medicines for a particular symptom, it may be difficult to know which one to take.

I once sent my husband on a trip with our toddler with a medicine kit for emergencies. I had filled it with generics but my husband didn't know which was which. He could not tell from the names on the bottles which was a decongestant, and which was an allergy medication.

What follows is a list of some of the medications with their brand names and generic names. It is only a guide. It is not a complete list. You should always go over your medicines with your doctors and follow their instructions. I recommend taking your medicine bottles with you to your visits to review the reason you are taking each medicine. Write the reason on the bottle with a marker so you can read it more easily than the printed labels. Keep track of when you need your prescriptions refilled.

Common Instructions:

PO=by mouth; IV=intravenous; PRN=as needed.

Long Acting=sustained release; steady effect; lasts longer.

Quick Acting=quick to start acting; lasts shorter time.

X=for number of times; for example x2 days=for 2 days OR x2=twice.

Brand Name	Generic Name	Reason to take	How to take OR as instructed
Anti Nausea Medications			
Compazine	Prochlorperazine	Nausea	PRN every 6 hours PO
Zofran	Ondansetron	Nausea	PRN every 6-8 hours PO
Aloxi	Palonosetron	Nausea	IV before and after chemotherapy
Emend		Nausea	PO, once before chemotherapy and once daily for 2 days after, in combination with Zofran and Decadron
Ativan	Lorazepam	Nausea, anxiety, sleep	Up to 3 times a day, PRN, PO
Decadron	Dexamethasone	Nausea, multiple uses	As instructed, 2-4 times a day.
Reglan	Metoclopramide	Nausea/ sluggish intestines, to increase motility	Up to 4 times daily, PO, PRN
Benadryl	Diphenhydramine	Nausea, allergy, sleep	Up to 3 times daily PO, PRN
Pepcid	Famotidine	Heartburn/ nausea	20 mg 1-2 times daily

Brand Name	**Generic**	**Reason to take**	**How to take OR as instructed**
Mouth Care			
Biostatin	Nystatin suspension	Thrush/ candida	Swish and swallow, 4 times daily
Lidocaine viscous		Mouth pain	Swish/ swallow PRN
Hydrogen Peroxide		Clean mouth debris	Rinse and spit PRN
Baking soda in warm water	Soda Bicarbonate	Clean mouth debris, help healing	Rinse and spit many times a day PRN
Kepivance	Palifermin	Mouth inflammation with high dose chemotherapy	IV for 3 days before and after chemotherapy
Constipation			
Senekot	Senna	Stool softener	1-2 pills 1-2 times daily
Colace	Docusate	Stool softener	1-2 pills daily
Miralax	Polyethylene glycol	Stool softener	Once daily, as instructed
Dulcolax	Bisacodyl	Stimulate bowel action	1-2 pills/ suppository, as instructed
Metamucil	Psyllium	Stool bulking agent	With water, as instructed.
Prune Juice		Stimulates bowel action	PRN
Mineral oil		Constipation	Single dose, PRN

Brand Name	**Generic Name**	**Reason to take**	**How to take OR as instructed**
Fleet enema		Constipation	Rectally, with caution during treatment, after instructions from your team.
Diarrhea			
Imodium	Loperamide	Control diarrhea	4 mg first, then 2 mg after each loose stool, max 16 mg/day
Lomotil	Diphenoxylate and Atropine	Control diarrhea	2 tablets 3-4 times daily PRN
PeptoBismol	Bismuth subsalicylate	Control diarrhea	2 tablets every 30 minutes, max 8 tablets, PRN
BRAT diet:	Bread, Rice, applesauce, tea	Control diarrhea	Avoid foods with high fat content.
Pain medications			
Motrin/Aleve	NSAIDs	Pain, inflammation	Use with caution during chemotherapy and with kidney disease
Tylenol/Anacin	Acetaminophen/ Paracetamol	Pain	No more than 4 gm daily. Use with caution with liver disease
Vicodin	Hydrocodone+ acetaminophen	Pain	Every 4-6 hours, PO, PRN. Monitor total acetaminophen dose per day.

Brand Name	Generic	Reason to take	How to take OR as instructed
Percocet	Oxycodone+ acetaminophen	Pain	Every 4-6 hours. Monitor total acetaminophen per day.
Oxycodone		Pain: quick acting	Every 4-6 hours PRN, PO
Oxycontin	Oxycodone CR	Pain: Long acting pain control	Twice daily, every day. Combine with quick acting medications as needed. Dose can be increased as needed.
Morphine		Pain: quick acting	Pills or liquid, as instructed
MS Contin/ Kadian	Morphine CR	Pain: Long acting	Once or twice daily depending on preparation. Combine with short acting as instructed.
Duragesic patch	Fentanyl	Pain: long acting	Change patch every 3 days. Dose can be increased for pain control. Combine with quick acting medication as needed.

NOTE: Most pain medicines can only be prescribed in limited amounts for limited durations. You will need a written prescription when you need a refill. Keep track of the medicines you may need to be refilled. Call your doctor's office by Thursday if you need a new prescription so they can provide it before the weekend. The on-call weekend doctor may not be able to give you a new prescription.

APPENDIX 3

3. Family History Tree

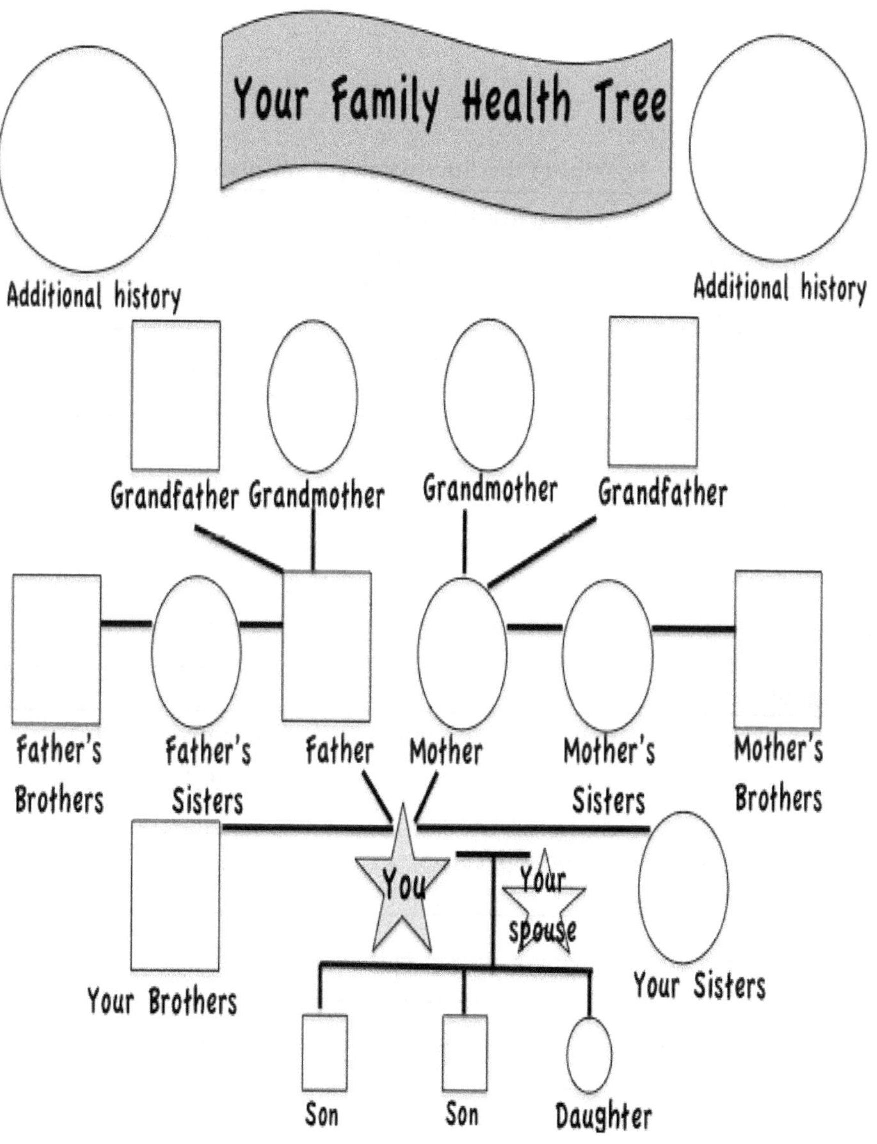

APPENDIX 4

4. Survivorship Care Plan

Format of the Survivorship Care plan:

General Information	
Patient Name:	Patient DOB:
Patient Phone:	Email:
Health Care Providers (Including Names, Institution)	
Primary Care Provider:	
Surgeon:	
Radiation Oncologist:	
Medical Oncologist:	
Other Providers:	
Treatment Summary	
Diagnosis	
Cancer Type/Location/Histology Subtype:	Diagnosis Date (year):
Stage: _I _II _III _Not applicable	
Treatment	

Surgery _Yes _No	Surgery Date(s) (year):
Surgical procedure/location/findings:	

Radiation _ Yes _No	Body area treated:	End Date (year):

Systemic Therapy (chemotherapy, hormonal therapy, other) _ Yes _No

Names of Agents Used	End Dates (year)

Persistent symptoms or side effects at completion of treatment:
_ No _ Yes (enter type(s)):

Familial Cancer Risk Assessment

Genetic/hereditary risk factor(s) or predisposing conditions:

Genetic counseling: _ Yes _ No
Genetic testing results:

Follow-up Care Plan

Need for Ongoing (adjuvant) Treatment for Cancer _ Yes _ No

Additional Treatment	Planned Duration	Possible Side effects

Schedule of clinical visits

Coordinating Provider	When/How often

<table>
<tr><th colspan="2">Cancer surveillance or other recommended related tests</th></tr>
<tr><td>Coordinating Provider</td><td>What/When/How Often</td></tr>
<tr><td></td><td></td></tr>
<tr><td></td><td></td></tr>
<tr><td></td><td></td></tr>
<tr><td></td><td></td></tr>
<tr><td colspan="2">Please continue to see your primary care provider for all general health care recommended for a person your age, including cancer screening tests. These symptoms should be brought to the attention of your provider:
• Anything that represents a brand new symptom;
• Anything that represents a persistent symptom;
• Anything you are worried about that might be related to the cancer coming back.</td></tr>
<tr><td colspan="2">Possible late- and long-term effects that someone with this type of cancer and treatment may experience:</td></tr>
<tr><td colspan="2">Cancer survivors may experience issues with the areas listed below. If you have any concerns in these or other areas, please speak with your doctors or nurses to find out how you can get help with them.
• Stopping Smoking
• Emotional and Mental health
• Physical Functioning
• Weight changes
• Financial Advice or Assistance
• Insurance
• School/Work
• Memory or Loss of Concentration
• Parenting
• Fertility
• Sexual Functioning
• Fatigue
• Other</td></tr>
</table>

Lifestyle/behaviors can affect your ongoing health. This includes the risk for the cancer coming back or developing another cancer. Discuss these recommendations with your doctor or nurse: • Tobacco use/cessation • Diet • Alcohol use • Sunscreen use • Weight management (loss/gain) • Physical Activity
Resources you may be interested in:
Other comments:
Prepared by: Delivered on:

APPENDIX 5

5. Screening for Cancer

Why Is screening necessary after a cancer diagnosis?

After completing cancer treatment, patients are watched carefully for any recurrence. In addition, all patients need to be vigilant for other cancers, because if you have had one kind of cancer, you may be at risk for another kind. Smokers who have been treated for throat cancer, for example, have to be screened for lung cancer.

It is important for cancer survivors to keep up with routine screening tests, and it is important for your family members to be correctly screened for cancer also. Depending on the cancer you had, your family's risk for cancer has now risen, and your cancer diagnosis needs to be added to each family member's medical record.

Common excuses to avoid screening procedures.

"My doctor keeps after me to have a colonoscopy. I don't want to go through that awful prep. Do I have to?"

"I don't feel bad, so why do I have to have that uncomfortable pelvic exam? I haven't had one for years, and I feel fine."

"I have blood work with my annual physical. Doesn't that find cancer?"

All cancers will eventually cause symptoms that will lead to diagnosis. Usually, as we presented in Chapter 2, by the time the symptoms cause you to seek medical attention, the cancer is at an advanced stage and more difficult to treat. Screening tests find cancer early, in a curable stage.

A Screening test is successful in saving lives if:

* **The disease is reasonably prevalent in the general population.** The test cannot find a needle in a haystack. If the disease is not common, screening large numbers of asymptomatic people to find early disease is not effective, and it is costly.

* **The test is relatively easy to administer and relatively inexpensive.** The test itself should be safe and carry no risk to people who do not have the disease. The general population would not accept a risky test. People who need to have a colonoscopy, for example, often avoid the procedure because they find the bowel cleansing preparation difficult to do, so there is an ongoing search for an easier screening test that will be more acceptable. If the test were very expensive, the cost to administer it to the general population would become prohibitive.

* **The test needs to be specific**. This means that if you test positive, the disease is truly present. You should not test positive if you don't have the disease. This is called a *false positive*, and it means that although your test is positive, there is no disease. A false positive test leads to unnecessary alarm and discomfort from additional procedures that ultimately do not find any Cancer.

* **The test needs to be sensitive.** It should not miss disease if disease is present. A negative test if you truly have the disease is a *false negative*.

* **Most important, screening is useful only if curative treatment is available at the early stage of diagnosis.** If there is no effective treatment at the early stages, when the disease is not causing symptoms, there might not be much benefit in diagnosing cancer.

Can blood tests for tumor markers be used as screening tests?

Tumor markers are not useful in early detection of cancer because they are not sensitive or specific enough. Tumor markers are proteins produced and shed by normal as well as abnormal cells, and they do not specifically diagnose cancer. As we discussed in the chapter on the pathology report (Chapter 5), tumor markers are useful to measure a patient's response to treatment in advanced cancer once that cancer has been diagnosed and treated. If the numbers are elevated at the time of diagnosis, watching the numbers go down is reassurance that the cancer treatment is working. If a patient's numbers are not elevated at the time of diagnosis, then the tumor marker is not useful to measure disease response or progression for that person.

Screening Recommendations compiled from the US Preventive Services Task Force and the American Cancer Society.

CANCER	TEST	WHO	WHEN (Years)	HOW OFTEN	STOP/NOT NEEDED
BREAST	Mammo-gram	If needed-- Universal--	40-44 45-54	Annually Annually	Life
					BUT
			54+	Every 1-2 years	Continue physical exams.
CERVIX	Pap smear		21-29	Every 3 years	
			30-65	Every 5 years	
			65+ with normal tests for 10 years.		Stop
			Total Hysterect-omy NOT Cancer related.		Does not need.
COLON	Colono-scopy OR Barium Enema OR Flexible Sigmoido-scopy	Family History will change age to start.	50-75	Every 3-10 years, depending on finding.	
			75-84	Consider	
			84 +		Does not need.
LUNG	Low dose Spiral CT Scan	Average Risk			Does not need

CANCER	TEST	WHO	WHEN (Years)	HOW OFTEN	STOP/NOT NEEDED
		High Risk: Active Smokers OR quit within last 15 years	50-74	Annually	15 years after quitting OR in poor health.

Screening tests are available for

- Breast Cancer: Mammograms.
- Cervical Cancer: Pap smears .
- Colon Cancers: Colonoscopy OR Sigmoidoscopy, stool testing for hidden blood, OR Barium Enemas.
- Lung Cancer in high risk populations only: Low Dose CT scans.

Prostate Cancer screening has been controversial. The PSA blood test has been widely used and has the ability to detect early stage cancer. However, there is controversy whether finding and then treating all prostate cancer early actually saves lives. Many of these cancers grow very slowly. If you find early stage prostate cancer in an elderly population, it may not need to be treated. Unfortunately, the screening test can lead to unnecessary, and sometimes uncomfortable, intervention. In its natural course this cancer may not have caused death, but the treatment for it can be harsh. Prostate cancer screening is beneficial in targeted situations.
At age 45: Screening is beneficial if your father or brother had prostate cancer before age 65 or you are African-American.
At age 50: Discuss pros/cons of testing for prostate cancer with your doctor. If you choose to be tested, use the PSA blood test and a digital rectal examination.

Screening is much desired but ineffectual in several cancers. One is ovarian cancer which doesn't cause symptoms until the disease is advanced. Screening with blood tests, e.g. CA 125, has not proven to be specific to cancer alone because it produces too many false positives. Pancreatic cancer is also silent in the early stages and is not common enough to warrant routine CT scans.

Until what age should you continue screening tests?

For example, Susan's grandmother has been going for mammograms well into her 90s. Now an abnormal calcification has shown up, and she is going to go through a biopsy and possible surgery for a condition that might not have grown in her lifetime or caused her discomfort or death. A physical exam and targeted evaluation of symptoms is sufficient at a certain age. Common sense should prevail.

NOTE: Many screening tests are being marketed directly to the consumer. They are not necessarily validated by strong data and may give you a false positive (tell you that you have cancer when you do not) leading to additional and possibly unnecessary invasive testing. A few years ago radiology companies offered whole body CT scans to look for "hidden cancers." Is one scan enough, or do you have to undergo annual CT scans to detect evolving cancers? How many cancers did this actually diagnose, and did it justify radiation exposure to an otherwise healthy population? When you hear of cancers being accidentally discovered in someone because of a scan they had for another reason, it is tempting to consider a "body scan," but this is not recommended to screen for cancer.

Action Plan

- Follow recommended screening guidelines.
- Practice risk reduction: Exercise, quit smoking, and improve your diet.
- Know your family history: It will have an impact on screening recommendations.

APPENDIX 6

6. Advance Directives

Examples of forms from the Commonwealth of Massacusetts.

1) Health Care Proxy designating your agent who will make medical decisions for you if you are unable to do so for yourself.

MASSACHUSETTS HEALTH CARE PROXY FORM

I, ____(the principal), residing at______________________________, ______________ County, Massachusetts, pursuant to Massachusetts General Laws Chapter 201D, appoint the following person to be my Health Care Agent:

Name: ______________________ Phone #: ______________________

Address:____________________ City/State/Zip: ________________

If my Health Care Agent named above is not available, I name as an alternate Health Care Agent:

Name: ______________________ Phone #: ______________________

Address:____________________ City/State/Zip: ________________

I give my Health Care Agent authority to make all health care decisions on my behalf if I become incapable of making such decisions for myself, including but not limited to decisions concerning initiation, continuing, withdrawing or refusing any life-prolonging care, treatment, service or procedure, EXCEPT (here list the limitations, IF ANY, you wish to place on your Agent's authority):

____

____

____

____

____

My Health Care Agent shall make health care decisions for me in accordance with my Health Care Agent's assessment of my wishes, including my religious and moral beliefs. If my wishes are unknown, my Health Care Agent shall make such decisions for me only in accordance with my Health Care Agent's assessment of my best interests.

My Agent may obtain any and all medical information, including confidential medical information, as I would be entitled to receive. Photocopies of this Health Care Proxy shall have the same force and effect as the original and may be given to other health care providers.

My Health Care Agent's authority to act on my behalf shall exist only for the period during which my attending physician determines that I lack capacity to make or communicate health care decisions for myself.

I sign this Health Care Proxy on ______________, 20_____ in the presence of two witnesses.

Signed:____

(If the Principal cannot sign) The principal is unable to sign and at the direction of the principal I have signed his/her name in his/her presence and in the presence of two witnesses.

Name:____

Street:____________________ City/Town: ____________________

2. Example of Advance Directives for Life Sustaining Treatment, obtained from the MOLST form in Massachusetts.

MEDICAL ORDERS FOR LIFE-SUSTAINING TREATMENT (MOLST) www.molst-ma.org
Patient's Name :
Date of Birth:
Medical Record Number if applicable:
A: check one circle
CARDIOPULMONARY RESUSCITATION: for a patient in cardiac or respiratory arrest
o Do Not Resuscitate o Attempt Resuscitation
B: check one circle
VENTILATION: for a patient in respiratory distress
o Do Not Intubate and Ventilate
o Intubate and Ventilate
o Do Not Use Non-invasive Ventilation (e.g. CPAP)
o Use Noninvasive Ventilation (e.g. CPAP)
C: Check one circle
TRANSFER TO HOSPITAL
o Do Not Transfer to Hospital (unless needed for comfort)
o Transfer to Hospital
PATIENT: mark who is signing
Section D:
o Patient o Health Care Agent o Guardian*
o Parent/Guardian* of minor representative
Signature of patient confirms this form was signed of patient's own free will and reflects his/her wishes and goals of care.
Signature by the patient's representative (indicated above) confirms that this form reflects his/her assessment of the patient's wishes and goals of care, or if those wishes are unknown, his/her assessment of the patient's best interests.

SIGNATURE: ______________________________
SEND THIS FORM WITH THE PATIENT AT ALL TIMES.

APPENDIX 7

7. Master Action Plan

Make Good Lifestyle Choices.

- Follow recommended screening guidelines.
- Listen to your body. Do not avoid reporting worrisome symptoms.
- Give your doctor feedback if the symptoms do not go away.
- Avoid cancer-causing habits, mainly tobacco use.
- Limit alcohol, fats, and red meat.
- Eat more fruits and vegetables.
- Exercise. Aim for normal BMI.
- Use antiviral vaccines when appropriate: Hepatitis, HPV.
- Know your family's cancer history.

As you are waiting for your Biopsy report, before Cancer is confirmed:

- Don't jump to conclusions. Wait until you get all your results.
- If the diagnosis is not certain, don't jump to a premature conclusion.
- Be aware that searches on the web may not provide accurate information.
- Do focus on a healthy lifestyle. Take care of your body.
- Exercise.
- Use alcohol in moderation.
- Quit smoking if you smoke.
- Eat a healthful, balanced diet.

- **Read this book to educate yourself**. Make notes as you go along.
- These lifestyle changes will help you whether your biopsy shows cancer or not.

When you get your Pathology report:

- Do not jump to conclusions. The initial biopsy report does not report the stage.
- If you read your pathology report, underline what you do not understand.
- Remember the technical words in the pathology report have different meanings than we understand in our common language.
- Write down your questions.
- Wait for your oncology consultation. Ask for an explanation.
- Gather your family history: Who was diagnosed and treated for cancer? What was their age at diagnosis? What kind of cancer was confirmed and (possibly) at what stage? What was the outcome?
- Gather your resources: Family, friends, neighbors, and co-workers who want to help.
- Be organized. Keep your records and an agenda book.
- Turn on your answering machine or voicemail.
- Turn off call blocking for unknown numbers. Your doctors' offices will be calling you. They need to be able to reach you.

During your consultations:

- Ask to record the consultation so you can go back and listen to the explanation.
- If a vital member of your family is not able to attend, ask if they can listen in on a speaker-phone connection in the room.
- Designate one person as a note taker and contact person.
- Update your contact information at the doctor's office.

Questions to ask.

- What is the stage of my cancer?
- What are my treatment options?
- What is the best treatment for my stage?

- What is the outcome with treatment? What is the outcome without treatment?
- Should I enroll in a clinical trial?

Where should you be treated?

- Verify that your local cancer center is certified.
- Verify that your local oncologists have the appropriate qualifications.
- Ask your local oncologists if they work with a specialty cancer Center.
- Ask about a second opinion. Ask who your doctor recommends.
- Ask if there is a patient navigator who can help you arrange the consultations.
- Weigh the pros and cons of where you are treated: Locally or at a specialty center.
- Find your own comfort zone.

Questions about Treatment Options:

- Ask which treatment is the standard first approach for your stage of cancer.
- If you have surgery, will you need any other treatments to improve the post surgical outcome? Radiation, chemotherapy, hormone therapy?
- If you have radiation or chemotherapy first, is surgery planned afterwards?
- If radiation therapy is part of a standard treatment plan, will you need chemotherapy simultaneously? Or later?
- Is chemotherapy the main treatment? How many treatments will you need?
- Can your cancer be treated with the new targeted therapy drugs?
- If you have metastatic disease, what are your treatment options? Would you be a candidate for surgery at a later point?

Preparing for Treatment:

- Clear your schedule for the appointments.
- Take someone with you for the teaching sessions.

- Ask to record the session so you can review the information.
- Can you get a flu shot?
- Can you have dental work?
- Ask about a Port.
- Ask about nutrition counseling.
- Can you exercise during treatment?
- Ask about infection precautions. Do you need to stay away from crowds?
- Can you work during treatments?
- Check with your employer's Human Resources department to see if you can take medical leave.
- Should you bring someone with you for the treatments?
- Is there any assistance with transportation?
- Order a wig if you need one.
- Get the prescriptions you need.
- Take help from friends and relatives.
- Ask for a referral to a fertility specialist if you need it. Consider whether there is adequate time to pursue fertility treatment before you start cancer therapy. Discuss fertility preservation options and decide whether they are right for you.
- Stay active and positive.
- Enquire about available support groups.
- Use your support systems: Family, community, workplace or religious affiliations.

Are you strong enough for treatment?

- Can you improve your performance status (or physical condition)?
- Do you need physical therapy?
- Do you need oxygen?
- Do you need pain management?

Nutrition Action Plan:

- If you need to, consult with the dietitian or speech & swallowing therapist.
- Maintain adequate nutrition and hydration.

- Clean, Separate, Cook, and Chill your foods carefully.
- Limit alcohol and caffeinated beverages.
- Continue with good dental care to avoid tooth decay and gum disease.

Exercise Action Plan:

- Consult a physical therapist if needed.
- Walk for 15 to 30 minutes daily, or as much as you can during treatment.
- Try Yoga or Tai chi for gentle muscle conditioning and balance.

Evaluate your Goals:

- Know the stage of your disease.
- Review the success rate of the recommended treatment.
- Discuss life expectancy and goals of treatment.
- Decide if the benefits of the treatment are in keeping with your life expectancy.
- Know your odds because they will guide your decision.
- Remember the odds are only a guide, not a certainty.
- Consider counseling.
- Complete your Advance Directives and Health Care Proxy instructions.
- Consult with hospice if you will not benefit from treatment.

Complementary and Alternative Therapies:

- Discuss your complementary therapies with your medical team.
- If you research unconventional medications, consider the source of the information. Discount the information if the source is the vendor who is selling you the medications.
- Ensure that any complementary therapy does not interfere with the recommended treatment.
- Use alternative therapies with caution.

Cancer Prevention:

- Limit Alcohol, Red Meat, and Processed Meat.
- Increase Vegetable, Fruit and Whole Grain consumption.

- Avoid Tobacco.
- Stay active. Exercise 30-60 total minutes daily.
- Consider a baby Aspirin daily.
- Consider available vaccinations.
- Limit Sun exposure.

APPENDIX 8

8. Glossary

ADLs: Activities of Daily Living measure the functional state of the person.
Advance Directives: Instructions you give in advance about the extent of life support or resuscitation measures you wish to undergo for yourself.
Anemia: Low Red Blood Cell count or low Hemoglobin in the red cell.

Biopsy: Sample of tissue taken from a suspicious site.
BMI: Body Mass Index is a measure of obesity.
BSA: Body Surface Area is calculated from height and weight and is used to calculate the dose of chemotherapy for each patient.

Cancer, Invasive: Cancer cell has penetrated natural boundary.
Cancer, In situ: Cancer cells within a defined lining layer.
Cancer, Grade: Degree of disorganization of nucleus.
Cancer cell Differentiation: Degree of similarity of cancer cell to cell of origin.
Chromosome: Organization of genetic material in the nucleus of the cell.
Clinical Trial: Stepwise approach (Phase 1, 2, and 3) to study new treatments.
Conference, Multidisciplinary Clinic: Patient is seen by different Cancer Specialists (Medical and Radiation Oncology and Surgery) in one setting.
Conference, Tumor Board: Conference involving different specialists who review scans and pathology without the patient present.
CBC: Complete Blood Count measuring your white cells, which fight infection, red cells, which carry hemoglobin, and platelet cells, which help to stop bleeding.

DNA: Special amino acids arranged in a specific sequence and formation on a chromosome which provide the building blocks of the genetic code.

FDA: Food and Drug Administration ensures the safety and efficacy of drugs and certifies quality control of drug manufacture.
Frozen Section: Quick look at the tissue from the site by the Pathologist during an operation.

Gene: A specific sequence of DNA that carries the genetic code.
Gene Mutation: A faulty gene or a change in gene or protein structure affecting function.
Gene Mutation, Dominant: Only one faulty gene of the pair is required for disease.
Gene Mutation, Recessive: Both copies of the pair need to be faulty in order to cause disease.

Health Care Proxy: Person/s you have designated to make medical decisions on your behalf in the event you cannot make them for yourself.
Hematologist: Doctor who treats blood disorders which can be a bone marrow cancer like leukemia OR disorders like anemia or bleeding and clotting disorders that are not cancers.
Hospice: Care provided to terminally ill patients to alleviate suffering.

Immunoperoxidase stains: Special dyes to help identify cells.
Infusion: Medicine mixed into a solution and put into your blood stream via a needle inserted into your vein.

Lymph node: Normal collection of cells along the lymphatic circulation that filter the lymph fluid and process immunity.
Lymph node, sentinel: Lymph node identified by dye injection to be first in the line of spread of cancer cells from the primary tumor.

Oncogene: Cancer-causing gene.
Oncologist, Medical: Doctor specializing in cancer treatment with chemotherapy, hormone therapy, targeted agents or immunotherapy.
Oncologist, Radiation: Doctor specializing in cancer treatment with radiation.
Oncologist, Surgical: Doctor specializing in cancer surgery.

Pathologist: Doctor specializing in identification of disease by examining cells.
Performance Status: measure of physical condition and functioning.
Primary Care Doctor: Family Doctor or General Practitioner.
Port/Portacath/VAD: A device placed inside your chest for intravenous infusion.

Radiologist: Doctor specializing in reading scans.
Radiologist, Interventional: Doctor specializing in performing biopsies under the guidance of scans and placement of ports or stomach tubes, for example.
Receptor: Special gateway protein on cell membrane.
Remission: Absence of visible disease.

Scans: Different radiological methods of examining internal structures, for example a mammogram, ultrasound, CT scan, MRI or PET scan.
Screening: Tests designed to detect cancer in its early, asymptomatic stage.
Staging: Determining extent of disease mapping all the locations of the disease.
Surgery, Curative: Removal of entire tumor and necessary surrounding area, leaving no cancer behind.
Surgery, Palliative: Surgery with intent of removing the portion of tumor that is causing local problems, for example blockage or bleeding.
Surgical Margin: Edge of the tissue removed during surgery.
Surgical Margin, Clean: No cancer cells at the edge.
Survival, Five Year: Percentage of patients who will be cancer free five years after diagnosis.
Survival, Overall: Length of time from diagnosis.
Survivorship: Long term issues resulting from Cancer and the treatment.

Therapy, Complementary: Supportive treatments to standard treatment to help alleviate side effects, for example Acupuncture, Yoga or Massage therapy.
Therapy, Alternative: Treatments instead of standard or recommended treatments.
Treatment, Adjuvant: Treatment recommended after the main treatment to improve cure rates.

Treatment, Curative: Treatment that will eradicate cancer cells completely.
Treatment, Definitive: Treatment that is the primary mode of cure.
Treatment, Neoadjuvant: Treatment that is given before the primary treatment to shrink the tumor and improve cure rates.
Treatment, Non-curative, or Life- extending: Treatment that will not cure the disease but will slow disease growth.
Treatment, Palliative: Treatment that intends to alleviate symptoms related to the tumor.
Treatment, Radiosensitizing: Low dose chemotherapy given with radiation therapy to improve the effectiveness of radiation therapy.
Tumor: Shadow, lump or mass that shouldn't be there.
Tumor, benign: Can grow, but does not spread to distant sites, or cause death.
Tumor, malignant (cancerous): Can grow, spread to distant sites and cause death.
Tumor Markers: Blood tests that can detect some proteins shed by cancer cells, for example: PSA for Prostate Cancer, CA-125 for Ovarian Cancer, CEA for Colon Cancer.
Tumor, Primary: Original site of tumor.
Tumor, Secondary or Metastatic: Site of tumor away from primary site.

Viruses: HPV= Human Papilloma Virus
EBV= Epstein Barr Virus

APPENDIX 9

9. Resources

1) American Cancer Society www.cancer.org,
Main office: 250 Williams Street NW, Atlanta, GA 30303

2) National Cancer Institute: www.cancer.gov
9609 Medical Center Drive, Bethesda, MD 20892-9760

3) National Institutes of Health: www.nih.gov
9000 Rockville Pike, Bethesda, MD 20892

4) National Comprehensive Cancer Network (NCCN): www.nccn.org
275 Commerce Drive, Fort Washington, PA 19034

5) LiveStrong Foundation: www.livestrong.org
2201 East Sixth Street, Austin, TX 78702

6) Susan G Komen for the Cure, originally Susan G Komen Breast Cancer Foundation:
www.info-komen.org

7) Academy of Nutrition and Dietetics: www.eatright.org

8) National Center for Complementary and Integrative Health: https://nccih.nih.gov

9) Global Cures Foundation: www. global-cures.org

10) USDA for dietary guidelines: http://cnpp.usda.gov/publications/dietaryguidelines/2010/policydoc/chapter3.pdf

11) LiveStrong Survivorship Care Plan available at http://www.livestrongcareplan.org/

12) Relaxation exercise for insomnia: https://sleepfoundation.org/insomnia/content/relaxation-exercise

13) Information on Complementary Medicince can be obtained at the website of the National Center for Complementary and Integrative Health (NCCIH) https://nccih.**nih**.gov/

14) Information regarding herbal and other supplements is available at:

- website of the Memorial Sloan Kettering Cancer Center in New York, NY https://www.mskcc.org/cancer-care/treatments/symptom-management/integrative-medicine/herbs

- website of the Mayo Clinic in Rochester, MN. http://www.mayoclinic.org/drugs-supplements

Notes

About The Author Dr. Gauri Bhide, M.D.

I am a Medical Oncologist and have had the privilege of taking care of Cancer patients for almost 25 years. I trained in Medical Oncology and Hematology at Boston University and the Boston Veterans' Administration Medical Center in Boston, MA, where I treated a variety of Cancers in a diverse population. I then practiced in community hospitals in the Boston area affiliated with the Dana Farber Cancer Institute and the Massachusetts General Hospital (MGH). As a member of the MGH Cancer Center, I cared for patients in their satellite offices and hospitals and participated in their multidisciplinary clinics, tumor boards, and clinical trial programs.

Since I had the opportunity to treat a variety of different cancers, my clinical experience became broad and varied. My work has taken me to urban, suburban, and rural areas where each has provided its own unique experience. It also gave me an appreciation of the challenges each setting presents to cancer patients and their caregivers.

I attended medical school in Mumbai, India, where my school was part of a

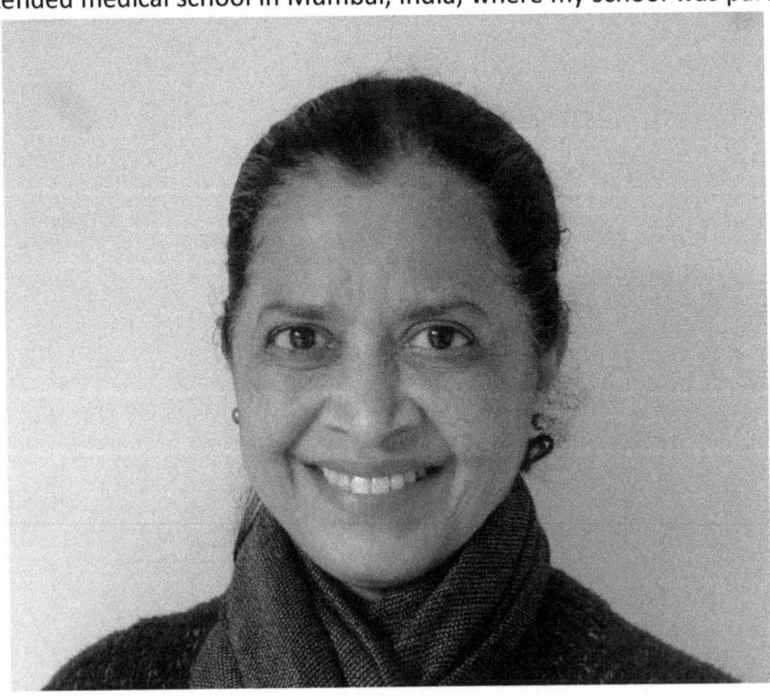

major hospital complex. The Tata Memorial Cancer Center down the street was the largest cancer center in Asia. My mother was a scientist at the premier Cancer Research Institute there, and her research was part of our dinner table discussions. She was involved in both laboratory and clinical research, and I saw how much passion she had for her work and how great the need was to improve patient treatment options and outcome. This resulted in my interest in cancer early in my medical career.

In addition to caring for patients, I have been a clinical advisor in a non-profit cancer research foundation called Global Cures. I am excited to participate in the Global Cures mission that has been to improve cancer treatment outcomes by re-purposing and re-discovering promising treatments and bringing them to clinical practice. I also serve as an advisor to other ventures that have a mission of improving survival in patients with cancer. I remain dedicated to the cause of patient education so that patients can participate with knowledge in their cancer treatment.

I live in the USA, in the Boston, MA, area with my husband and two sons. We enjoy tennis, travel, adventure, friends, and family.

Acknowledgements

Over many years of Oncology practice, patients and their families have inspired me with their fortitude. Friends and family members who have faced a cancer diagnosis have given me insight into what patients hear during their consultations and the questions that linger after they leave the doctor's office.

I am indebted to my husband, Michael, who patiently supported me with his time, his feedback, and encouragement. My sons, Vikas and Vishal, were self-sufficient when they needed to be and provided fun and distraction at other times. My thanks to my brother, Amar, who first suggested writing this guide and kept reminding me to make the time to do it.

Many friends gave generously of their time to read my drafts. Andrea Brand, Diane Krause, and Gay Bailey provided invaluable feedback. Robin Romero performed a yeoman's job in editing the manuscript, both in cleaning it up and sticking to my tight schedule. Skye Wentworth helped with her expertise in marketing.

Thank you all of you for helping me bring this book to publication.

Gauri Bhide, M.D.

Index

CPSIA information can be obtained
at www.ICGtesting.com
Printed in the USA
BVHW041929011221
623025BV00025B/569

9 780998 367316